Mental Health in East Asia

This pioneering monograph examines how culture informs popular understandings and experiences of mental health in East Asia, as well as provides resolutions for the future.

Questions about mental health problems have gained new urgency as their consequences are growing more visible in East Asia. Yet, our understanding, funding, and evidence have not kept pace. Anson Au explores the social and psychological concepts, and network structures that make up the blueprint of East Asian cultures and untangles their myriad influences on how people think, feel, and trust with respect to mental health experiences. Chapters explore themes such as cultural beliefs about mental health, the role of social support and social media, and mental health stigma.

Drawing on the latest quantitative evidence, network science, and novel qualitative data, this book paints a portrait of mental health in the region and articulates culturally sensitive policies and practices tailored for East Asian cultures that improve mental health experiences.

Anson Au, PhD, is Assistant Professor of Sociology at the Hong Kong Polytechnic University. An award-winning author of over forty scientific articles, he is an expert sociologist on economic sociology, social networks, digitalization, and professions and organizations, with a regional focus on East Asia.

Mental Health in East Asia

Cultural Beliefs, Social Networks, and Mental Health Experiences

Anson Au

Routledge
Taylor & Francis Group
NEW YORK AND LONDON

First published 2023
by Routledge
605 Third Avenue, New York, NY 10158

and by Routledge
4 Park Square, Milton Park, Abingdon, Oxon, OX14 4RN

Routledge is an imprint of the Taylor & Francis Group, an informa business

Library of Congress Cataloging-in-Publication Data
A catalog record for this title has been requested

ISBN: 9781032310374 (hbk)
ISBN: 9781032312415 (pbk)
ISBN: 9781003308720 (ebk)

DOI: 10.4324/9781003308720

Typeset in Sabon
by Apex CoVantage, LLC

For Robert Au, Florence Yuen, and Lo Mo-Lan.
謹以此書獻給區紹昌，袁桂芳，和盧慕蘭。

Contents

Preface

This monograph has been a long time in the making. It is an homage to my professional origins for I started my career in mental health. I went on to become a scholar of economic sociology and networks, and some of my insights in these respects have been integrated into this monograph to cast new light on mental health. But as rewarding as this professional cross-pollination has been, the motives for my foray once more in the subject of mental health were more human than they were professional.

The sight of friends fallen by their own hand is a force powerful enough to stir even stone from stasis to motion – to hope.

Mental health is a rare subject with universal pull. It is where we are confronted with mortality, ruin, and meaning with a capital "M" in all the ways we live, for the most compelling stories of mental health that haunt us are of loss, a lingering facet of life that appears to be rent from time and borders, surviving the premodern world to extend into the modern one.

Despite the universality of mental health, there remains an indigeneity that patterns its experience and renders it the province of culture. This monograph thus sets out to unpack the ways that this is true: how culture is a mental blueprint with which we understand life and at the same time whose dimension lines may be bars of a cage.

I hope that future generations will learn of mental health as love, rather than loss – that our hands will not grow so used to holding shovels that they forsake how to hold one another. In that spirit, this monograph came to be from much love, in the broadest and purest of senses.

I first thought about mental health, as I am sure most people do, before realizing the word. My brush with mental health began with my mother, father, and grandmother, whose struggles as immigrants impressed upon me the limits and purity of the human yearning for hope. The depths of their experience remain an abyss into which I can only peer and feel as existentially small as I do enormously grateful.

I also thank Scott Schieman, Stephanie Nixon, Cathy Cameron, Blair Wheaton, Bill Magee, Bonnie Erickson, Markus Schafer, and Fedor Dokshin at the University of Toronto, whose work and tutelage were formative for my understanding of social structure and mental health in the early years of my career.

I thank Rob Haddow and Tse-Chueen Chan at the South China Morning Post for their intrepid editorial work and guidance over the many years I have worked with the Post.

I thank Ben Ku, Eric Chui, Elise Yan, Jenny Chan, Karita Kan, Rodney Chu, Judy Siu, David Shum, Luke Fung, and Chi-tat Chan at the Hong Kong Polytechnic University for their support, friendship, inspiration, and guidance.

I also thank Ty Shin, Malak Al Tibi, Zhiheng Chen, Joseph-Christian Guittard, Stephanie Taing, Darrell Hosford, with whom I have discussed ideas in this monograph in some form. The conversations we shared remain a foundational part of myself.

I thank Ilho. May you be where words may yet be heard and where stardust dances in your soul as much as when you were here.

This monograph partly draws upon and rewrites excerpts of my past work in the *International Journal of Mental Health* by Taylor and Francis, the *European Journal of Mental Health* hosted by the Semmelweis University Institute of Mental Health, the *Bulletin of Science, Technology, & Society* by Sage, and the *South China Morning Post*. The journal articles in question are Au, A., & Chew, M. (2017), "How do you feel? Managing emotional reaction, conveyance, and detachment on Facebook and Instagram," *Bulletin of Science, Technology & Society*, 37(3), 127–137, DOI: 10.1177/0270467618794375; Au, A. (2017), "The sociological study of stress: An analysis and critique of the stress process model," *European Journal of Mental Health*, 12(01), 53–72, DOI: 10.5708/EJMH.12.2017.1.4; and Au, A. (2017), "Low mental health treatment participation and Confucianist familial norms among East Asian immigrants: A critical review, *International Journal of Mental Health*, 46(1), 1–17, DOI: 10.1080/00207411.2016.1264036.

1 Invigorating the Role of Culture in Mental Health

A Looming Crisis

A crisis is brewing in East Asia. Under the duress of exams amid a high-pressure environment, a student leaps without wings from the high perch of an apartment, a skyscraper, a school. The name escapes us, but the act presses into our memory with a morbid normalcy. An alarmingly consistent string of suicides has threaded through China, South Korea, and Japan.

In the cold hours of the evening on December 17, 2017, when the sun began to desert the sky, Kim Jong-hyun left into the gathering dark. Kim Jong-hyun was the lead singer of SHINee, a favorite among my generation, and the face of Korean pop's global influence at the peak of its popularity. More than idols, SHINee was an icon of an industry, bringing newfound attention to a country we'd scarcely heard of but would valorize for years to come. Yet, Jong-hyun perished in solitude, slunk against the walls of a rented apartment and bloated with the fumes from coal lit on a pan. Leaving carefully laid suicide notes in advance with close friends, he cited a long-standing fight with depression that devoured him as the reason for departing this world. The world stood still in the entertainment industry. For all the status he had accrued, for all the talent he possessed that we admired, all the money and fame he had earned, it wasn't enough. And for all the shock we feel, Jong-hyun was but the latest addition to a haunting legacy lingering among the halls of fame.

And a host of others we remember or have forgotten. Behind smiles and closed doors, the victims all passed without warning; all of them devoured and defeated by a shadow stalking around the dark. Money couldn't protect them. Nor fame. Nor even the adoration of millions across the globe. The suicide rates per capita for East Asian countries are the highest in the world. In South Korea, the male suicide rate stands at 32.5 for every 100,000, the third highest in the world, and that among females is 15 for every 100,000, *the* highest in the world. In Japan, suicide is the highest cause of death among men aged 20 to 44. Likewise, in China, Taiwan, and Hong Kong, suicide never stays away from the

DOI:10.4324/9781003308720-1

public eye for too long before students or workers seek a radical retreat from the demands of their work.

The names on our list of heartbreaks grow without regard for age. Pressing into our minds with morbid normalcy, they present different characters of the same tale. With every remake, the shock lessens, but the pain deepens. And in the silence of our breaths held, we are confronted with the question we dare not ask, yet feel under our skin: who's next?

So many have fallen. A silent majority suffers still. Though visceral, suicide is the result of a long, tortuous battle waged out of sight – and it's not the only outcome. Mental health problems are a process of falling that we don't see, but should.

The most insidious poisons are those that linger the longest. With infections strewn across East Asia, the coronavirus has bludgeoned the region's public health defenses. Pundits have rightfully turned their attention to how to curb the pandemic, but they seem to assume that everything will return to normal after it passes.

This cannot be further from the truth. We are faced with a deeper crisis unleashed by the pandemic, whose effects will be felt long after COVID-19 fades: a mental health crisis.

Having studied stress for years, I have observed that it is perhaps one of the most significant, yet most underestimated plague in modern societies. Stress is a matter of life and death. It is a precursor of mental disorders, like depression and suicide ideation, and diseases of despair, like alcoholism and substance abuse. Stress also indirectly increases the risk of major heart diseases and all-cause mortality, an effect that can begin as early as childhood (Johnson et al., 2020).

Mental health disorders are on the rise in East Asia. More and more workers in China report depression and anxiety each year. High-profile Korean celebrities have succumbed to personal pressure, blips in South Korea's suicide rate that sits among the highest in the world. More died in Japan by suicide than by COVID-19 last year. Millions still suffer in silence.

Figure 1.1 schematically breaks down the incidence rates of major mental health disorder in East Asia, or essentially how many new patients are reported with a given mental health disorder out of 100,000 people, from 2000 to 2019. The figure includes depressive disorders, drug use disorders, eating disorders, mental disorders, self-harm, and substance use disorders.

Depressive disorders include major depressive disorder, dysthymia, bipolar disorder, and anxiety disorder. Drug use disorders include opioids, cocaine, amphetamine, cannabis, and other drugs. Mental disorders include depressive disorders, schizophrenia, eating disorders, autism, attention-deficit disorder (ADD), conduct disorder, developmental intellectual disability, and other mental health disorders. Eating disorders include anorexia and bulimia.

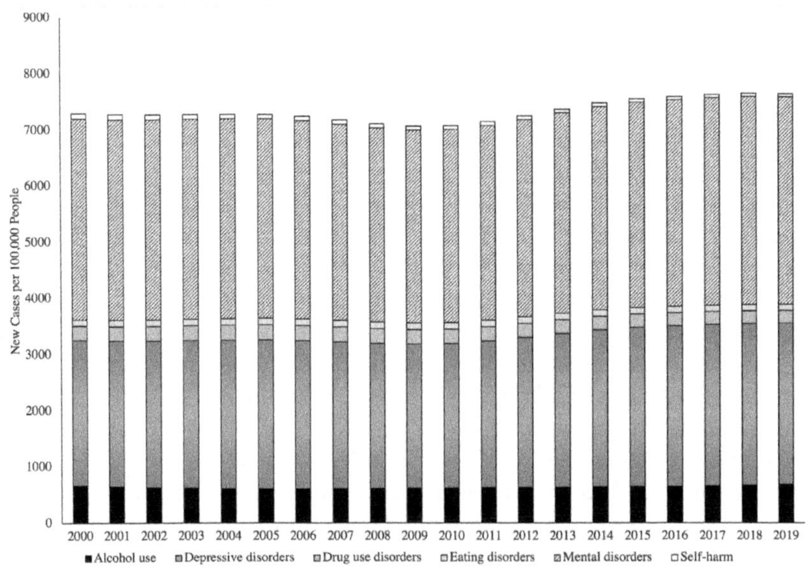

Figure 1.1 New cases of mental health disorders in 100,000 people in East Asia (2000–2019).

Source: Global Burden of Disease Collaborative Network (2020)

Over this 20-year period, some disorders appear to have eased up. Self-harm dropped in half from about 99 new cases in 2000 to about 55 in 2019. Drug use disorders have also edged down 10% from about 256 new cases in 2000 to 228 by 2019. But we should not overinterpret these two measures, since they were among the smallest disorders in scale to begin with.

The remainder and majority of disorders have increased during these past 20 years. Alcohol use edged up from 662 new cases in 2000 to 684 by 2019. Eating disorders largely held steady at 110 new cases during this period. Depressive disorders shot up by a staggering 10% from 2590 new cases in 2000 to about 2869 by 2019, a remarkable increase given that it was the largest disorder in scale to begin with. Along with it, mental disorders in general rose from 3580 new cases in 2000 to 3694 by 2019.

Even more worrying, stressors have only grown in number and magnitude, and stress has continued to reach all-time highs in the time that I have studied it. And with it, mental disorders have grown in kind. As Figure 1.1 shows, the incidence rates of new cases of mental health disorders like depression have largely notched new heights or retained their ground. When we turn to the prevalence of mental disorders (not pictured), the picture grows bleaker, with nearly every major disorder hovering around the same rate or increasing over the past decade.

Mainland China has begun taking steps to address this burgeoning crisis of stress and mental health, discussing safeguards against imposing limits on working hours in job sectors notorious for overwork like information technology (Feng, 2021). Yet, other modernized societies in the region very visibly trail behind. For far too long, the financial hardships, job precarity, and inequality that aggravate stress have been left completely unfettered.

The pandemic has exacerbated these existing stressors. Taking Hong Kong as an example, the latest wave has come to infect nearly 20% of Hong Kong's total population and will likely cause a range of long-lasting health problems on patients, as new issues emerge (Heung, 2022). What's more, the pandemic is bringing unprecedented job disruptions and spells of unemployment to hundreds of thousands of workers in nearly every job sector, but most of all the retail, service, and tourism sectors (Cheng & Ting, 2022). This hammer-blow to people's financial wellbeing will last for years, even after the COVID-19 pandemic ends.

Stress, mental health disorders, and other diseases are now a coiled spring ready to explode after the pandemic. Already, there are signs that residents are cracking. An October 2021 poll of secondary school students by the Federation of Youth Groups found that half of the students reported record level stress and showed signs of depression (Low, 2021). Not long after, a string of suicide attempts has now come to rock the city as quarantine and lockdown measures ramp up (Whitehead, 2022). Our best public health science tells us to expect more of the same, including higher levels of stress in the Hong Kong population and with it, greater prevalence and incidence rates of mental health disorders and health issues in general.

The costs are clear if governments in the region do not act now. The health and mental health repercussions of stress will lower health expectancy and overburden domestic healthcare systems. And as quality-of-life in the region falls, the size, talent, and integrity of the regional workforce will be compromised and, by extension, so will the very economies that are often cited as a source of pride.

The gravity of this crisis urges a fresh look at mental health. Let us turn to review the two major schools of thought about analyzing mental health: the stress process model and social determinants of health.

What Is the Stress Process Model?

The stress process model was created by Leonard Pearlin and colleagues in the latter half of the 20th century (Pearlin et al., 1981; Pearlin, 1983), and has since become a widely influential theory in the health and social sciences, informing tens of thousands of studies since its conception.

The starting point of the stress process model is the idea that every individual is inevitably immersed in a social environment comprised of his or her memberships in a plethora of different social settings that require interaction with others, such as family, work, friends, and so on. Stress, therefore, occurs when the relationship between an individual and his or her environment suffers from a lack of congruity, defined by Aneshensel (1996) as a state of arousal resulting from the presence of socio-environmental demands that tax the ordinary adaptive capacity of the individual or from the absence of means to attain sought-after ends. Thus, stress is not a fundamental characteristic of any number of conditions, but arises from dissonance between conditions and an individual's ability to adapt to them.

The stress process model is a theoretical framework that examines the causes and manifestations of stress, the intervention of resources that moderate and mediate stress, and the consequences of stress on an individual in terms of mental health and social adversities. This section outlines what the dynamics of the stress process are, at the same time critiquing its usage and highlighting gaps for future research. Given the rise of mental health studies purporting to apply the stress process model, this section articulates a more updated, foundational version of the model that includes key developments to its structure.

Stress and Stressors: An Introduction to Scale and Duration

The conditions from which stress can develop are called stressors. Stressors challenge our ability to adapt to a situation (Aneshensel, 1996) and often require us to adjust our behaviors in some way (Thoits, 2011). This is essentially how we feel stressed by something.

The stress process model breaks down stressors in terms of five major types and three different levels at which they can operate. The five major types of stressors exist along a continuum between being continuous (occurring on a long-term basis) and being discrete (occurring once or on a short-term basis): chronic, traumatic, nonevents, daily hassles, and life events (Wheaton, 1994; Wheaton et al., 2013). The three levels on which stressors can operate are micro, meso, and macro. Micro refers to exposure on personal levels. Stressors on any level can still be experienced by or affect an individual and translate to a form of personal stress, one that is internalized and responded to with a personal, emotional reaction.

Stressors are classified in the stress process model based on where they fit in terms of type and level. For example, discrimination is a stressor that can be considered continuous and divorce is a stressor considered discrete. Visible minorities faced discrimination in the job market and were segregated to lower-paying heavy labor jobs in America in much of the 1900s. Partners experiencing a divorce are traumatized, but their divorce happens once and never again. These examples also reflect stressors on the micro-level, things that are experienced in everyday life.

Scholars typically categorize stressors as either discrete or chronic (Brown et al., 2020; Wheaton, 1994; Wheaton et al., 2013), but as you might have surmised, they need not exist in a binary – they can often be both discrete and continuous. Daily hassles are a good illustration of this fluidity. Misplacing belongings or encountering traffic problems are daily hassles that might easily discrete and continuous. Even if traffic jams happen once or twice in your working day, you might well have to slug through traffic every day, especially if you live far away from work.

This fluidity is not just true of the micro-level – it also holds true in meso- and macro-levels. Meso refers to situations delimited by social boundaries like networks and communities. Exemplar stressors are neighborhood crime, something that is more chronic, and natural disasters, something more discrete. These stressors do not just strain an individual – they strain their entire community or network as well.

Macro refers to issues concerning larger political entities, such as states and nations. Within this level are the stressors affiliated with a larger system, including economic recessions, something more chronic, and nation-level crises like the September 11 attacks, something more discrete.

As these examples show, the rubric of types and levels in the stress process model are not as rigid as scholars typically assume. They are fluid. This fluidity is theoretically important to recognize because it opens up what we can do empirically; it sensitizes us to the theoretical idea that one stressor can actually cause or "spillover" into another, which opens up a whole new realm of study.

Stressors especially susceptible to this "spillover" are life events and trauma, defined by circumstances of a severe situation – like victimization in sexual assault. Though victimization in sexual assault or a divorce is initially discrete in the event's singular occurrence, it can easily percolate into an emotional scar or memory that constitutes a continuous stressor. The interconnectedness highlighted in this example further illustrates the potential causal relationships between stressors, such as trauma becoming chronic (Wheaton, 1994).

Another type of stressor is nonevents. Lack of change can be as stressful as change. Nonevents refer to stressors caused by the lack of something, such as the absence of favorable conditions or of goal attainment. Role captivity, explained later, is an example of this, where a person is not necessarily dissatisfied with their current position but with their inability to obtain a higher goal (Wheaton et al., 2013). Nonevents can also be likened to anticipatory stressors, where the expectation of something that has not or may not even happen causes stress. Thus, following the example of a sexual assault victim, the chronic stressor of an emotional scar can become a nonevent stressor through resilient fear of the recurrence of rape regardless of its likelihood.

The final type of stressor is also the most wide-ranging and complex: chronic stressors. Chronic stressors are those that exist on a long-term basis in an individual's life or ongoing difficulties. Wheaton (1997) classifies seven forms of chronic stressors: (1) perceived threat; (2) structural constraints – lack of access to opportunity to achieve ends; (3) underreward – relational deprivation where outputs are disproportionately lower than inputs or in contrast with others giving the same level of input; (4) uncertainty – the desire to have a conclusion when an outcome is not possible yet; (5) conflict that is regular and without resolution; (6) demands – when expectations cannot be realized with available resources; and (7) complexity – number of sources of demands or clash of responsibilities across roles.

The blueprint of these seven types of chronic stressors is consistently the presence of aversive socio-environmental conditions or the absence of benign socio-environmental conditions, which may include the absence of means for fulfilling aspirations (Brown et al., 2020). Dressler (1988) identifies three major types of environment-individual discrepancies that are part of this chronic type of stressor: status (disparity between occupation and income), goal-striving (disparity between aspiration and actual accomplishment), and lifestyle (disparity between consumption behavior and social class). These three types of discrepancies represent the presence of aversive conditions that prevent individual happiness, reflected in structural barriers inhibiting upward mobility. For example, a worker with an uncompromising manager may be drawn into a status discrepancy if he/she is assigned continual job enlargement (i.e., an expanding variety of tasks) without a similar addition reflected in his/her income.

What Causes Stress? The Role of Roles

Having reviewed how to think about stressors, we are led to ask: what causes stress? The stress process model recognizes that discrete stressors are by and large unpredictable. Life events like divorce, the September 11 attacks, or sexual assault are good examples. But chronic stressors are a different story. Chronic stressors were defined in the previous section as the presence aversive conditions or the absence of benign conditions. The stress process model has a specific way of viewing these conditions – through the idea of social roles. From our families to our friend circles, to our workplaces, to our extracurricular groups, we are assigned roles in every major domain of our social lives.

Roles are important because they reflect structural aspect that facilitates the stress caused by events and because of their enduring nature (Pearlin, 1983; Fu & Chen, 2021). That is, since roles themselves are long-term involvements, so too would be the stress that affects them. Even life events that are discreet can cause stress by altering the role of an individual, possibly creating a chronic type of stressor. For example, job loss can cause stress for an individual, but it may be more prominent if experienced by one who bears the role of a parent. In this instance, the role of parenthood intensifies the stress from job loss about the parent's responsibility to provide for his/her children and family. Furthermore, people attach notable importance to roles and their activities (McLeod, 2012; Pearlin et al., 1981), as they are socialized to devote themselves to institutional roles that contribute to society's maintenance. Such is the case with enduring roles like those related to families, occupation, economy, and education (i.e., parenthood, marriage, work). Thus, it is difficult for a person to remain apathetic to stress from within their roles or to that which affects their roles.

Roles also reflect larger contexts in which they are located, offering insight to social arrangements. We glean an example in occupational roles, where the consequences of arrangement, values, and social status in an organization are revealed through how people are affected by their jobs. The theoretical purchase of viewing roles as *contexts* calls attention to social status, which exists not only as an attribute of the individual but can be conceptualized as part of a deeper social inequality across different levels and types of hierarchy (Aneshensel, 2010; Wheaton & Clarke, 2003).

The Exceptional Qualities of the Family: A Critique

On that note, I offer a critique of conventional assumptions about roles by suggesting the exceptional qualities of the family as a space where stress is experienced that has not received enough attention in the stress process model (Au, 2017). First, it can be a major source of problems themselves, such as those found in marital or parent-child relations. Second, it is also the location where external problems are shifted to. Third, it serves as the environment in which people relieve their strains. While this idea highlights the family's distinct position, one point of critique on this idea is that it assumes the case of a heterosexual nuclear family. The popularity of the nuclear family is declining, being replaced by trends of common-law relationships and fewer children (Popenoe, 2020). The appeal of the common-law relationship is in the financial and work autonomies given to each member, where the responsibilities of domestic chores are not administered to women, but divided by negotiation (ibid.). Thus, either member of a common-law relationship share in a sense of equity, reducing the onset of problems experienced in marital relations related to finance or work. Same-sex unions may also fall into this pattern, being without gendered perceptions of roles and responsibilities, and which have grown over the years to now accounting for 0.82% of all couples (Statistics Canada, 2011). The growing diversity of families includes long-distance families that would also be less likely to align with the three dimensions Pearlin (1983) suggests, for example where distance prevents access to the physical family, making it less likely to be a place where problems could be transplanted or resolved.

Role Strain

When we experience hardships or problems through our roles, they become a source of stress for us or *role strains*. There exist six types of role strains in the stress process model (McLeod, 2012; Repetti & Wang, 2017):

(1) *Problems between an individual and the nature of a role's tasks.* Here the intervention of personal attributes is emphasized. Strains that appear objective actually involve a subjective evaluation component. Stress from work required for a job, for example, is actually dependent on interpretation. Work assigned by others can become role overload, characterized by an overload of work that is not self-chosen, but imposed by others (Pearlin, 1983, 1989). A point of critique in response to this is the weighted focus on subjectivity. If stress experienced by an individual not only depends on different factors but on an innumerable amount of them, then it must be asked whether stress can even be studied. If the stress of each person depends on too many things, then a study of stress should be untenably complex as it points to a plethora of possible routes that cannot be mapped.

However, this is not the case. Patterns can be established between the subjective and the objective. Socioeconomic status is a clear example of this, where disadvantaged people consistently encounter more strenuous circumstances that cause more stress than advantaged people due to lack of access to mediator resources and cultural capital (Mirowsky & Ross, 1999). Thus, as much as subjective interpretations are relevant, there is a correlation between objective conditions and stress (mediated by subjectivity) that represent predictable trends which offer insight to the sources of stress and to potential solutions for them.

(2) *Interpersonal conflict.* This type of strain arises from the relations between people involved in the same role set. Some examples of how this strain manifests include unequal effort being committed to something, disagreements in values, breakdown in communication, and depersonalization through absence of appreciation or acknowledgment (McLeod, 2012). Considering disagreement in values, personal values factor into the arousal of strain via their translation into conflicting practices. This is evident in the case of alienation in a workplace, in which it occurs with those who disagree with supervisors and exhibit low obeisance. The disconnection in values leads to segregation in the workplace.

(3) *Role captivity.* In this a person experiences a discrepancy between his/her current role and a desired one, facilitated through lack of means. It should be noted that the strain arises not from dissatisfaction with current roles but from the desire to be something else (Pearlin, 1983).

(4) *The loss and gain of roles that demands adaptation.* Gaining a role entails adaptation that may be strenuous, such as having a child and becoming a parent. Following this example, however, the strain from the acquisition of new roles may be mitigated by pre-socialization or preparation for it with classes and learning about child-rearing. Losses can be more commonly sudden, as with divorce or involuntary job loss, which encompasses trauma or transitions that cause significant stress. Pearlin (1983) accredits this to a lack of anticipatory socialization. An argument of critique on this, however, is that anticipatory socialization may actually shape existing relations and affect the outcome of certain contexts. Expectations of a divorce, for example, may influence a spouse's behavior, creating paranoia over trivial events or causing a decrease in the amount of effort invested (the mentality that 'it's going to end anyway') that may impact his/her partner and marriage. Thus, the outcome may be influenced by anticipatory socialization, becoming a self-fulfilling prophecy.

(5) *Role restructuring.* This is brought about involuntarily or with redistribution of status, privilege, or influence and is therefore more stressful than simply gaining or losing roles. A notable example deals with aging and the subsequent shift in responsibilities and behaviors as parents become cared for by their children. Autonomy and reliance are reversed: where the parent was once in charge, the child has now taken over the responsibilities and authority of caretaking. Thus, both parties may become stressed by the change in personal values as their roles become restructured. This point lends itself to underscore a point of critique, the changing nature of stressors in consideration of factors like aging (Pearlin & Bierman, 2013). The stressors a young person experiences are associated with performance in school and finding jobs. That is not to say, despite the lack of recognition, that these roles and their stressors are constant, for they will obviously change over time. Hence, the nature and the identity of a person's stressors both change as he/she ages, constituting role transitions as well as role restructuring.

(6) *Multiple roles and intrapersonal conflict.* Participation in multiple roles may create strains as demands from each collide. Contagion can also be observed within the multitude of roles a person is involved with (Pearlin, 1983). Stress can be proliferated via direct or indirect experience in roles. On the point of direct experience, strains in one role (a job) may stimulate more strains in another role (a marital role). The introduction of technology has further thinned the borders that once segregated a person's social life. For example, communication technologies increasingly enable the expansion of interactions between work and family life where one role's demands can project onto another, a phenomenon called role-blurring (Glavin et al., 2011) or spillover to address the lateral extension of stress across roles (Thoits, 1995;

Pearlin & Bierman, 2013). Furthermore, a role is often integrated as part of a role set that allows for indirect proliferation (Pearlin, 1983). For example, an occupational office role requires interaction with other roles like administration, clients, staff, and so on. Hence, problems in one of these would translate into problems for others, constituting another avenue in which stress can be proliferated.

How Does Stress Proliferate?

How else does stress proliferate? Stress does not necessarily require direct exposure by a person to be effectuated. It may be transmitted through interaction with social environment and the subsequent projection of problems onto the self. In the example of a rape victim, the stress that a rape victim feels is anticipatory, characterized by fear of precedence or by an event in the future that has not happened or may not happen (Fanfan et al., 2020). Individuals often feel stressed in anticipation of events in everyday life, such as when their fear of crime rises following a criminal act inflicted on someone within their social networks or even broader neighborhood (Agnew, 2002; O'Brien et al., 2019). On a larger or macro level, the similar proliferation of anticipatory stressors is assumed by Pearlin and Bierman (2013) to be observable in economic conditions and effects on citizens, where financial strains learned through media (i.e., the hardships associated with recessions) stimulate fear for personal economic outlooks.

This is similar to how stress can be acquired through others via a contagion effect (Aneshensel, 2010). Stress is often not restricted to a single individual but imposes on others around them. This contagion effect is more prominent in the context of families where people experience the effects of stress encountered by those emotionally close to them. Coyne and associates (1987) examined spouses of two groups of depressed patients, where one was in recovery. Though they found that spouses of the two groups were stressed for different reasons, both were stressed regardless and not free from hardship. Their results shed light on the nature of the contagion effect in terms of stress, where stress in one person leads to that in others. Research decades later has continued to corroborate these ideas (Repetti & Wang, 2017).

Stress proliferation can also occur across roles in the forms of role-blurring or spillover as previously explained, such as when a spouse finds that the demands of care-giving for patients take away from or interrupt other domains of life.

What Resources Do People Use to Adapt to Stress and Stressors?

How do we adapt to stress and stressors? The stress process model suggests that while a person's social conditions and subjective proclivities may be stressors, they could also be tools for mitigating stress. *Resources* are thus things that are drawn upon in reaction to stress, with the quality of reducing the impact of stressors (Thoits, 1995, 2011). However, the nature of the effect of resources can be variable. For instance, resources may affect the impact of stressors in a beneficial manner (called moderating the effect of stressors) or be themselves influenced by stressors to aggravate the situation (such as when stress spreads from one spouse to another). A resource is not confined to be either positive or negative but rather depends on circumstances. There are four resources that stand out: coping, social support, mastery, and belief systems (Pearlin & Bierman, 2013; Wheaton et al., 2013).

Coping

Coping has been the most extensively studied resource, which is a cognitive response to a stressor that prevents the harm caused by it. Pearlin and Bierman (2013) outline possible functions, including avoiding or eliminating the stressor, preventing stress proliferation (secondary stressors), altering the meaning of a situation, or confining the emotional impact. With the case of coping resources, avoidance is one such example of the point mentioned earlier on the ambivalence of resources. Avoidance is useful for reducing the impact of short-term stressors and generally produces positive psychological outcomes (Taylor & Stanton, 2007), but in a long-term context, avoidance could translate to emotional suppression, where frustration builds up to a point of aggravated release. For example, while coping resources are effective in moderating stressors, a form of coping that alleviates personal stress can cause strain in others. A spouse's choice of avoidance may lead to detached behavior that impacts his/her spouse and their relationship. Furthermore, the social conditions for which resources work differ, such as the discovery of how coping resources, are more effective in the workplace than with individuals (Chung, 2018).

Social Support

Social support refers to the functions performed for a person by significant others and is divided into three categories by House and Kahn (1985): emotional, informational, and instrumental. Found to be inversely proportional to psychological disorders, within these three types of social support are the satisfaction of one's emotional and social needs for affection, identity, security, and assistance (Au, 2019). Hypotheses for this pattern include the assumption that social support imparts a sense of mattering, where one's identity is important to someone else (Pearlin & Bierman, 2013). A person consequently feels comforted with a sense of identity and of an emotional bond of affection. Another possibility is the legitimating effect of social support that reaffirms the validity of a person's choices, or the validity of their feeling stressed. Support from others conveys confidence in identity and esteem, reassuring the person that the stress they experience is reasonable per the circumstances and is not the product of personal defects (Pearlin & Bierman, 2013; Thoits, 2011). Yet another potential reason is the actual effect caused by others, where the influence of others has a visible impact on a person's lifestyle or values that mitigate disorders. As outlined by Thoits (1995), social support resources in the form of emotional support have been found to directly correlate with mental health and buffer the impact of stressors. It is best measured by the existence of an intimate relationship where greater intimacy means greater efficacy (i.e., spouse or lover is stronger than friendship).

The Stress of Social Support: A Critique

I note that there is an understudied nuance to social support as a resource. Stress process model scholars recognize that social support resources, like all resources, may be depleted over time (Brough et al., 2018). A person's social group may find the person annoying and distance themselves from him/her, lowering the insulation that this social support would normally provide against stressors. This idea opens up a point of critique of the stress process model: more than simply becoming an ineffective resource, social support might actually become a stressor itself.

Reduction in social support may not only represent the growing absence of a mediator but the growing presence of a stressor. While assumptions are commonly made that a person who steadily loses friends is simply more exposed to the original stressors, this presumes that this person is indifferent to this loss. In other words, this trend of losing friends itself may become an actual new stressor for the person through the act of self-attribution (Aneshensel, 1996, 2010), such as ruminating on self-depreciative thoughts like "why am I so pathetic that I lost my friends?" This self-prescribed trait of being pathetic could then cause the person to retreat from seeking social support, heightening the deleterious effects of the original stressors.

Three further points should be noted: first, social support resources may not be used even if available. For instance, males usually do not have as strong ties with a social circle as females do, per societal norms surrounding a man's image of independence and strength (Webster et al., 2018). Second, in light of a previous point of critique on the change in stressors caused by aging, an adherent point of critique holds that any likewise alterations in available resources must also be recognized. As a person ages, the nature of their resources changes in addition to that of their stressors. This is particularly evident in the case of social support, where a person's social circles and connections diminish over time as they age, causing a subsequent drop in availability of social support resources. Children also become part of the social support that is available to aging parents, further underlining the role reconfiguration in the inversion of dependence and autonomy between children and parents in the process of aging.

Lastly, just as a person's coping resources can be detrimental to others (as with the example of someone becoming more avoidant in his marriage, thereby affecting his spouse), so too can social support resources cause more problems for others. A person may choose to draw from a form of social support that in itself is problematic by nature. Participation in a subculture that endorses illicit activities, for example, creates disorder on a larger scale. The appeal of a deviant subculture is in the creation of a domain that allows for new opportunities to obtain the prestige, recognition, and satisfaction which a person might not otherwise receive in other areas of life (Blackman, 2014). For example, a person could join a drug-user or gang community to achieve a sense of escapism or empowerment, regardless of any damage to the larger community.

Mastery

Mastery refers to the individual perception of ability to handle stress. A common variable affiliated with mastery is socioeconomic status, where the higher a person's socioeconomic status is, the more education and occupational background and prospect he/she would have, and consequently the higher his/her sense of mastery (Schieman & Plickert, 2008) would be. Thus, personal control may at times be less associated with individual characteristics and more with availability of privileges in higher statuses (Pearlin & Bierman, 2013). It should be emphasized that this positive correlation between mastery as a resource and socioeconomic status is shared by all moderating resources (Fanfan et al., 2020; Mirowsky & Ross, 1999) simply due to the advantageous background a higher socioeconomic status affords that better facilitates progression in society than a lower one (i.e., better education, better job prospects, more finance for endeavors).

There are four ways in which mastery is assumed to lessen the effect of stressors: first, the threat from particular stressors is perceptually minimized or neutralized, second, the reduced threat contributes to a sense of self-confidence in abilities to overcome the stressors (Pearlin & Bierman, 2013). Third, mastery has been found to encourage social learning and flexibility that improve the probability of effective behavior rather than escape behavior in addition to learning to prevent the occurrence of stressful events (Frögéli et al., 2019). Lastly, it is indicated that a sense of control reduces the impact of stressors via promoting problem solving in their consequences (Pearlin et al., 1981).

Resources, like stressors, are not independent of one another. Green and Rodgers (2001) write that social support resources influence and are influenced by mastery. Their studies following low-income Black mothers revealed that social support resources can add to a person's sense of self-efficacy, where higher perceived support contributed to higher self-efficacy and less perceived stress. The reverse was also found to be true. Higher self-efficacy led to perceived higher social support, thereby enabling people to actually reach out and establish this social support. Connections can therefore also be made between other resources, such as a greater sense of control (self-efficacy) leading to better coping strategies. For example, a person believing in their own power to influence the situation may create more confidence to manage their emotions.

The Stress of Mastery: A Critique

I offer another critique of the stress process model's ideas of mastery here. A sense of control in moderation may be beneficial for the reasons described earlier. Having a low sense of control could make people more vulnerable to stressors, where a person believes he/she is incapable of overcoming the stressor and thus not only is impacted more in terms of mental health but also stops putting effort into resolving problems, believing in a fatalistic future (i.e., 'if I'm going to fail anyway, why should I try?').

But we do not always know our own limits. So, at what point does mastery become delusion? Put differently, having too much mastery could establish the conditions for deleterious effects. When a person with a high sense of control encounters a stressor beyond the scope of his expectations, the impact is suddenly more intensified than it would be for a person with a lower mastery. For instance, a person who firmly believes in the stability of his/her job would face more trauma and require more adaptation to a job loss than a person who wanted or expected to quit anyway.

Belief Systems

Beliefs may be an important buffer for stress. Belief systems comprise hierarchical systems of values and meanings, such as religions. A hierarchical system of importance can help assuage the effect of stressors through a misalignment between reality and perceived importance. In religion, faith and devotion to ritual may lower the potency of a stressor such as when a religious worker loses their job, believing that God has something better in store for them. Under religious determinism, a person is reassured that everything is planned and will be good, leading him/her to more willingly strive to overcome stressors.

The Stress of Belief Systems in East Asian Cultures: A Critique

An additional critique on the topic of resources and much of the stress process model is the lack of focus on non-Western cultures like in East Asia. Most of the research done has been conducted under the premise of a Western culture assumed to be inherently understood by and manifested in individuals.

What about East Asians? A belief system can amplify the effects of stressors if important values and adverse conditions align. For instance, in East Asian cultures, education is heavily emphasized. A student who receives a poor grade thus experiences even *more* stress because of their belief systems.

Belief systems may also work against a person's benefit by stifling the enactment of coping resources. Koreans, for instance, do not readily seek out mental health support from fear of the stigma associated with it by their culture, to be discussed later (Au, 2017). Belief systems may thus limit the visibility – and accessibility – of social resources in the first place.

What Are the Effects of Stress?

Single and Multiple Outcomes

What does stress do? In the stress process model, stressors challenge adaptive capabilities, causing strenuous experiences that inflict damage to mental, well-being, behavioral, and/or social aspects. Thus, stress arises when this strain is internalized by a person, whereby the damage or disorder it inflicts can be measured by a study of its psychological, physical, and behavioral manifestations, and their influence on how people live their lives (Pearlin, 1989).

Psychological consequences of stress most commonly refer to mental health outcomes. These are all possible consequences, where stress eventually erodes or is unaffected by available resources (Nagy et al., 2020). If a person is unable to manage stress, he/she may suffer from a loss of confidence, identity, affection, and sense of control. Through this, he/she may be led to believe he/she is alone, unwanted or unimportant, and incapable of overcoming difficulties or succeeding. Such thoughts, characterizing the traits of anxiety, anger, and depression (Pearlin & Bierman, 2013), can translate into a frustration towards the self and surrounding social conditions and can thrust people into a stasis of unhappiness made perpetual not only by their circumstances but also by their emotional responses.

Much focus of stress research has been dedicated to single-outcome studies of the social antecedents of mental health problems (Aneshensel, 1996; Pearlin & Bierman, 2013). It should be noted that, as some researchers have pointed out previously, the act of equating mental health effects of stress with specific disorders may misrepresent the power of stressors and of group differences in reaction to stress, while shifting the concentration of stress outcomes disproportionately to mental health in neglect of other areas.

What About Physiological Consequences? A Critique

In addition to psychological consequences, there are also physiological ones. Physical consequences of stress follow a pattern of physiological alertness and exhaustion. Stress process model scholars have criticized this as lacking in the necessary considerations of context, experience, and social ramifications (Wheaton et al., 2013). However, their critique does not deny the existence of a physiological or even psychological impact but rather illustrates the importance of the social aspects of stress. Furthermore, the biological response to stress is constant. For example, whether a person suffers a breakdown from a divorce, an uncompromising boss, or a bankruptcy, the breakdown entails the same chemical and hormonal responses regardless of the source of stress.

Recent groundbreaking research shows that being stressed is and can *become* genetic. An innovative field called epigenetics has shed light on the "nature" versus "nurture" debate by showing us that genetics and health consequences are shaped by both. A prominent article published in *Nature*, the foremost scientific journal in the world, shows that the health behaviors, practices, and consequences we glean from our environment ("nurture") actually become built into our genes as we continue living (Zannas & Chrousos, 2017). Some early evidence of this comes from addiction studies dealing with alcohol and tobacco abuse, which have shown that addictions are passed down. But more recently, scientists are discovering that the stress we experience in real life actually functions in the same manner. Stress changes our genes to make us more predisposed to being stressed. Just as important, this stress tendency becomes passed down.

Thus, despite the importance of the psychological and social, the effects of stressors go beyond mental health consequences to include physiological ones. Both must be assessed in conjunction with the social aspect, for while these two constituents are important, they cannot be allowed to overshadow the higher-level social framework of the roots and indications of stress and stressors that sets the stage for analyses on lower levels.

What Are Social Determinants of Health?

The social determinants of health school of thought are similar to the stress process model. The social determinants of health paradigm begins with the recognition that social factors play an enormous role in shaping our health. Although it has traditionally focused on general and physical health, recent work has brought the social determinants of health idea into understanding mental health as well. This section outlines what the main argument is and the most common social determinants that have been studied in this idea.

Upstream and Downstream Social Determinants of Health

The social determinants of health school of thought is commonly thought of as a river. Imagine a river that people living in a nearby village drink from. Imagine also that after some time, the villagers fall ill and show signs of poisoning. To understand why these villagers fell sick, we can take a downstream view and an upstream view. A downstream view looks at the most immediate factors that make a person ill. In the case of the river poisoning, we might look at the fact that people drank from the river in the first place. An upstream view looks further – at the more distant, yet fundamental causes of illness. Tracing the toxins flowing in the river, we might encounter upon a factory upstream pumping industrial waste into the river.

Thinking in terms of upstream and downstream matter for the solutions that we come up with for health problems more generally. In the river example, a downstream solution might be distributing filters for the villagers to purify river water prior to drinking. An upstream solution, however, would focus on fixing the fundamental source of the toxins, like closing the factory upstream or managing its waste distribution program. The social determinants of health school of thought focus on upstream factors.

Upstream Determinants

Upstream determinants that affect mental health have to do with the social structures or broader patterns associated with social attributes. Such attributes include, for example, educational attainment, socioeconomic status, gender, and race or ethnicity. These attributes work by affecting our life chances or, rather, the social and economic resources that we will have access to over the course of our lives both directly and indirectly.

Social determinants affect our resources directly. Higher educational attainment has a strong effect on our ability to get a job, later ability to rotate into new jobs, and how much money we'll be paid over the course of our working lives (Braveman et al., 2011). In multiracial societies that are increasingly the case in a globalizing world, inequalities similarly surface across different genders, classes, and racial or ethnic groups. Women consistently face disadvantages and verbal abuse in the workplace, as do those belonging to racial or ethnic minority groups (Karlsen & Nazroo, 2002).

Upstream determinants also exert indirect effects on our social and economic resources. Sociological research has found that educational attainment provides unspoken forms of cultural resources. Going through years of university education socializes us to etiquette about how to behave in professional settings, something that pays off tremendously in the job market. Studies have examined these differences between immigrants and natives of a given society, where immigrants suffer disadvantages as early as in the job hiring process by failing to understand interview etiquette (Nee & Sanders, 2001).

Just as important, it isn't only educational attainment that affects this kind of cultural resource. Race or ethnicity and class play similar roles as well. Children of parents who do not have postsecondary education or who belong to lower socioeconomic classes, with lower household income, report facing similar challenges in the workplace (Fernández-Kelly, 2008; Manevska & Achterberg, 2013). Without having early role models or instructors to socialize them into the cultural etiquette of professional work, many face being locked out of higher-paying jobs. Thus, the poor, in essence, end up staying poor.

Social and economic resources, in turn, shape our health by determining our standard of living. How much income or financial assets we have at our disposal very evidently factor into every choice we make about our living conditions. Having low income might mean a family needs to live in neighborhoods that have poor air or water quality and remains close to facilities that manage hazardous waste, much like the village example. The structure of the residences that a family needs to live in itself might be old, increasing exposure to lead paint, mold, pests, or so on (Sallis & Glanz, 2006). The surrounding neighborhood might also be unsafe, predisposed to higher rates of violence, accidents, or crime and lack the resources for exercise, such as sidewalks or parks (Heinrich et al., 2007). Such neighborhoods might then create more distrust in inhabitants, which deprives them of the ability to seek out social support and to live happily without anxiety (Williams & Collins, 2001). A low-income family might also be forced to choose to live in residences farther from the city core where jobs are most densely clustered, increasing the amount of time they spend on commutes and, by the same token, minimizing the time they can spend on leisure, family, and non-work-related activities (Diez Roux & Mair, 2010).

Working conditions is also an important upstream determinant of our health. Low-income families and minorities are siphoned into menial labor roles that often feature unsafe working conditions and exposure to hazardous materials. In a global environment of rising corporatization and deunionization, these workers are further disadvantaged with fewer protections against wage stagnation, loss of employee benefits, and strenuous working hours (Neumark et al., 2012).

Income is a powerful upstream determinant. It can introduce constraints in our education, living conditions, and working conditions. It also affects what foods we can afford, the medical care we can afford when we get sick, and so on. This, essentially, is how inequalities of class and ultimately health come to replicate themselves.

What Are the Consequences of Social Determinants of Health?

The social determinants of health school of thought orients us to focus on the long-term consequences of any social factor. Like in the river example, some of these toxins can linger in the body for a long time, at the same time affect entire households, neighborhoods, or even societies. A toxic river affects multiple generations of villagers, coming to fundamentally reshape the course of their lives.

Poor life circumstances affect our health and mental health. The danger, according to the social determinants of health school of thought, is that the reverse is also true. Poor mental health comes back to constrain life chances. Differences in wealth between rich and poor households show up in childhood development, which goes on to affect psychological development, educational attainment, and adult health – and the cycle repeats when these adults have children of their own.

Upstream social determinants like education, living conditions, housing conditions, and class outlined prior thus prefigure health and mental health outcomes at every stage of life. Deprivation of economic resources needed to survive is a tremendous, chronic stressor that stays with people through the life course. Social determinants also shape our mental health by indirectly affecting social resources outlined in the stress process model, such as social support and sense of mastery or control over our own lives. In a large-scale study of adolescents in the United States, Finkelstein and colleagues (2007) find that adolescents whose parents had a higher education felt less stressed than those whose parents did not. In particular, adolescents whose parents had lower educational attainment were ultimately less engaging, less optimistic, and, therefore, more stressed and less able to cope as a result. In a telling survey of Canadian workers, Koltai et al. (2018) similarly find that once people move below the low-income threshold, they feel much more anger. While personal sense of mastery can reduce the amount of anger that people feel, this downward mobility itself can reduce the amount of mastery and control that people feel about their life circumstances. This is consistent with a large amount of evidence that demonstrates that lower socioeconomic class weakens mental health and mastery (Ross & Mirowsky, 2013).

Toward a Cultural Turn in Mental Health

The stress process model and the social determinants of health are adept frameworks that enable the mapping of stress on multiple levels. They provide an interpretive understanding of stress in different contexts and under the influence of different domains. But there's another truth to this picture, hidden in the rising tide of mental health issues in East Asia: mental health is cultural – the main argument of this book.

This cultural view is missing from the major schools of thought that examine mental health. Culture does not consist merely the objects we consume but the infrastructure of our very modes of thought: the unwritten values, norms, and schemas that become baked into the way we structure our institutions, relationships, and roles. The cultural rules that order our lives thus similarly come to mediate our experience of mental health.

In the chapters that follow, I map out how this transpires in the context of East Asia. Chapter 2 discusses the architecture of prototypical East Asian culture: the core beliefs that order social life in the region and how they inform unique meanings of mental health, wellness, and illness. This chapter breaks down these cultural beliefs into an overarching orientation toward communitarianism, through which arise the concepts of communal belonging and obligation to familial honor that order individual decisions. This chapter articulates how these concepts filter perspectives toward mental health, wellness, and illness as complications of the individual's ability to fulfill familial obligations.

Chapter 3 examines how culture informs stigma toward mental health, with a critical eye on the stereotypes about mental health. It will also assess how social networks are the bedrock social unit that embeds people in East Asian cultures and how they accordingly facilitate the contagion of stigma and how they are ultimately transformed by stigma itself.

Chapter 4 examines the social resources that help people cope with mental health in East Asia. The social network structures outlined in Chapter 3 are brought to bear on the nature of trust and social exchanges in East Asia, which tend to be expressive with kinship ties, but rationalistic with non-kinship ties. I assert that this arrangement is a double-edged sword: on the one hand, it invigorates socializing, but on the other, it discourages much-needed emotionality.

Chapter 5 discusses how East Asian culture affects the demand and delivery of professional services. Drawing connections between themes raised in the previous chapters (beliefs about wellness, stigma, coping, and social support), I theorize that stigmatized beliefs about mental health come to shape professionals' own beliefs about mental health potentially for good, in terms of developing culture-specific strategies, and for bad, in terms of biases and the discouragement of mental health service.

Chapter 6 investigates the role that social media plays in shaping mental health in East Asian cultures in an age of digitalization. I discuss the ways that technical features of social media are synergizing with cultural etiquette to offer relief for mental health – by making people more open to emotions – but also worsen mental health by spreading addiction and personal information through networks.

In the conclusion, I briefly highlight the most common stressors as they apply to East Asia, including trends in income inequality, education, health care, and the labor market. I discuss how the social psychological concepts and social network structures of East Asian culture build atop these stressors to amplify deleterious mental health consequences. I conclude by proposing culturally sensitive policies and practices tailored for East Asian cultures that aim to improve mental health experiences in grassroots, institutional, and clinical settings, and ultimately legitimize mental health.

References

Agnew, R. (2002). Experienced, vicarious, and anticipated strain: An exploratory study on physical victimisation and delinquency. *Justice Quarterly*, *19*, 603–632.

Aneshensel, C. (1996). Consequences of psychosocial stress: The universe of stress outcomes. In H. B. Kaplan (Ed.), *Psychosocial stress: Perspectives on structure, theory, life-course, and methods* (pp. 111–136). New York, NY: Academic.

Aneshensel, C. (2010). Neighborhood as a social context of the stress process. In W. R. Avison, C. Aneshensel, S. Schieman, & B. Wheaton (Eds.), *Advances in the conceptualization of the stress process* (pp. 35–52). New York, NY: Springer.

Au, A. (2017). Low mental health treatment participation and Confucianist familial norms among East Asian immigrants: A critical review. *International Journal of Mental Health*, *46*(1), 1–17.

Au, A. (2019). The embodiment of social capital at individual and communal levels: Action, rewards, inequality, and new directions. *International Journal of Sociology and Social Policy*, *39*(9/10), 812–830.

Blackman, S. (2014). Subculture theory: An historical and contemporary assessment of the concept for understanding deviance. *Deviant Behavior*, *35*(6), 496–512.

Braveman, P., Egerter, S., & Williams, D. R. (2011). The social determinants of health: Coming of age. *Annual Review of Public Health*, *32*, 381–398.

Brough, P., Drummond, S., & Biggs, A. (2018). Job support, coping, and control: Assessment of simultaneous impacts within the occupational stress process. *Journal of Occupational Health Psychology*, *23*(2), 188–197.

Brown, L., Mitchell, U., & Ailshire, J. (2020). Disentangling the stress process: Race/ethnic differences in the exposure and appraisal of chronic stressors among older adults. *The Journals of Gerontology: Series B*, *75*(3), 650–660.

Cheng, L., & Ting, V. (2022). Coronavirus: Hong Kong has no plans for 'wholesale city lockdown', leader Carrie Lam insists, as record 55,000 new covid-19 cases confirmed. *The South China Morning Post*. Retrieved from www.scmp.com/news/hong-kong/health-environment/article/3168912/coronavirus-hong-kong-private-hospitals-should

Chung, Y. W. (2018). Workplace ostracism and workplace behaviors: A moderated mediation model of perceived stress and psychological empowerment. *Anxiety, Stress, & Coping*, *31*(3), 304–317.

Coyne, J., Kessler, R., Tal, M., Turnbull, J., Wortman, C. B., & Greden, J. (1987). Living with a depressed person. *Journal of Consulting and Clinical Psychology*, *55*(3), 347–352.

Diez Roux, A., & Mair, C. (2010). Neighborhoods and health. *Annals of the New York Academy of Sciences*, *1186*, 125–145.

Dressler, W. (1988). Social consistency and psychological distress. *Journal of Health and Social Behaviour*, *29*, 79–91.

Fanfan, D., Rodríguez, C., Groer, M., Weaver, M., & Stacciarini, J. (2020). Stress and depression in the context of migration among Haitians in the United States. *Health & Social Care in the Community*, *28*(5), 1795–1806.

Feng, C. (2021). Big Tech's excessive 996 overwork culture in China is illegal without extra compensation, top court reminds employers. *The South China Morning Post*. Retrieved from www.scmp.com/tech/tech-trends/article/3146662/big-techs-excessive-996-overwork-culture-china-illegal-without

Fernández-Kelly, P. (2008). The back pocket map: Social class and cultural capital as transferable assets in the advancement of second-generation immigrants. *The Annals of the American Academy of Political and Social Science*, *620*(1), 116–137.

Finkelstein, D. M., Kubzansky, L. D., Capitman, J., & Goodman, E. (2007). Socioeconomic differences in adolescent stress: The role of psychological resources. *Journal of Adolescent Health*, *40*(2), 127–134.

Frögéli, E., Rudman, A., & Gustavsson, P. (2019). The relationship between task mastery, role clarity, social acceptance, and stress: An intensive longitudinal study with a sample of newly registered nurses. *International Journal of Nursing Studies*, *91*, 60–69.

Fu, Y., & Chen, J. (2021). The influence of parental migration on left-behind children's mental health in China: The mediating roles of daily stress and sense-making. *Applied Research in Quality of Life*, 1–23.

Glavin, P., Schieman, S., & Reid, S. (2011). Boundary-spanning work demands and their consequences for guilt and psychological distress. *Journal of Health and Social Behavior*, *52*, 43–57.

Global Burden of Disease Collaborative Network. (2020). *Global Burden of Disease Study 2019 (GBD 2019) results*. Seattle, WA: Institute for Health Metrics and Evaluation (IHME).

Green, B., & Rodgers, A. (2001). Determinants of social support among low-income mothers: A longitudinal analysis. *American Journal of Community Psychology*, *29*, 419–440.

Heinrich, K., Lee, R., Suminski, R., Regan, G., Reese-Smith, J., Hugh, H. H., Haddock, K. C., Carlos Poston, W. S., & Ahluwalia, J. S. (2007). Associations between the built environment and physical activity in public housing residents. *International Journal of Behavioral Nutrition and Physical Activity*, *4*, Article 56.

Heung, S. (2022). Coronavirus: Why Hongkongers recovering from Covid-19 at home feel helpless and frustrated. *South China Morning Post*. Retrieved from www.scmp.com/news/hong-kong/health-environment/article/3168937/coronavirus-why-hongkongers-recovering-covid-19?module=lead_hero_story&pgtype=homepage

House, J., & Kahn, R. (1985). Measures and concepts of social support. In S. Cohen & S. L. Syme (Eds.), *Social support and health* (pp. 83–108). New York: Academic.

Johnson, J., Chaudieu, I., Ritchie, K., Scali, J., Ancelin, M. L., & Ryan, J. (2020). The extent to which childhood adversity and recent stress influence all-cause mortality risk in older adults. *Psychoneuroendocrinology*, *111*, 104492.

Karlsen, S., & Nazroo, J. Y. (2002). Relation between racial discrimination, social class, and health among ethnic minority groups. *American Journal of Public Health*, *92*(4), 624–631.

Koltai, J., Bierman, A., & Schieman, S. (2018). Financial circumstances, mastery, and mental health: Taking unobserved time-stable influences into account. *Social Science & Medicine*, *202*, 108–116.

Low, Z. (2021). Hong Kong pupils showing signs of depression as new school year brings heavier workload and added stress. *The South China Morning Post*. Retrieved from www.scmp.com/news/hong-kong/health-environment/article/3154589/hong-kong-students-showing-signs-depression-new

Manevska, K., & Achterberg, P. (2013). Immigration and perceived ethnic threat: Cultural capital and economic explanations. *European Sociological Review*, *29*(3), 437–449.

McLeod, J. (2012). The meanings of stress: Expanding the stress process model. *Society and Mental Health*, *2*, 172–186.

Mirowsky, J., & Ross, C. (1999). Economic hardship across the life course. *American Sociological Review*, *64*, 548–569.

Nagy, E., Moore, S., Silveira, P. P., Meaney, M. J., Levitan, R. D., & Dubé, L. (2020). Low socioeconomic status, parental stress, depression, and the buffering role of network social capital in mothers. *Journal of Mental Health*, 1–8.

Nee, V., & Sanders, J. (2001). Understanding the diversity of immigrant incorporation: A forms-of-capital model. *Ethnic and Racial Studies*, *24*(3), 386–411.

Neumark, D., Thompson, M., & Koyle, L. (2012). The effects of living wage laws on low-wage workers and low-income families: What do we know now? *IZA Journal of Labor Policy*, *1*(1), 1–34.

O'Brien, D. T., Farrell, C., & Welsh, B. C. (2019). Looking through broken windows: The impact of neighborhood disorder on aggression and fear of crime is an artifact of research design. *Annual Review of Criminology*, *2*, 53–71.

Pearlin, L. (1983). Role strains and personal stress. In H. Kaplan (Ed.), *Psychosocial stress: Trends in theory and research* (pp. 3–32). New York: Academic.

Pearlin, L. (1989). The sociological study of stress. *Journal of Health and Behavioural Science*, *30*, 241–256.

Pearlin, L., & Bierman, A. (2013). Current issues and future directions in research into the stress process. In C. Aneshensel, J. Phelan, & A. Bierman (Eds.), *Handbook of the sociology of mental health* (pp. 325–340). New York: Springer.

Pearlin, L., Lieberman, M., Menaghan, E., & Mullan, J. (1981). The stress process. *Journal of Health and Social Behavior*, *22*, 337–356.

Popenoe, D. (2020). *Disturbing the nest: Family change and decline in modern societies*. London: Routledge.

Repetti, R., & Wang, S. W. (2017). Effects of job stress on family relationships. *Current Opinion in Psychology*, *13*, 15–18.

Ross, C., & Mirowsky, J. (2013). The sense of personal control: Social structural causes and emotional consequences. In C. Aneshensel, J. Phelan, & A. Bierman (Eds.), *Handbook of the sociology of mental health* (pp. 379–402). New York: Springer.

Sallis, J., & Glanz, K. (2006). The role of built environments in physical activity, eating, and obesity in childhood. *Future Child*, *16*, 89–108.

Schieman, S., & Plickert, G. (2008). How knowledge is power: Education and the sense of control. *Social Forces*, *87*, 153–183.

Statistics Canada. (2011). *2011 Census of Canada: Conjugal status and opposite/same-sex status (7), sex (3) and age groups (7A) for persons living in couples in private households of Canada, Provinces, Territories and Census Metropolitan Areas, 2011 census*. Retrieved Mai 20, 2016, from http://www12.statcan.gc.ca/census-recensement/2011/dp-pd/tbt-tt/Rp-eng.cfm?LANG=E&APATH=3&DETAIL=0&DIM=0&FL=A&FREE=0&GC=0&GID=0&GK=0&GRP=1&PID=102574&PRID=0&PTYPE=101955&S=0&SHOWALL=0&SUB=0&Temporal=2011&THEME=89&VID=0&VNAMEE=&VNAMEF=

Taylor, S., & Stanton, A. (2007). Coping resources, coping processes, and mental health. *Annual Review of Clinical Psychology*, *3*, 377–401.

Thoits, P. (1995). Stress, coping, and social support processes: Where are we? What next? *Journal of Health and Social Behaviour*, 53–79.

Thoits, P. (2011). Mechanisms linking social ties and support to physical and mental health. *Journal of Health and Social Behavior*, *52*, 145–161.

Webster, J. R., Adams, G. A., Maranto, C. L., & Beehr, T. A. (2018). "Dirty" workplace politics and well-being: The role of gender. *Psychology of Women Quarterly*, *42*(3), 361–377.

Wheaton, B. (1994). Sampling the stress universe. In W. Avison & I. Gotlib (Eds.), *Stress and mental health: Contemporary issues and prospects for the future* (pp. 77–114). New York: Plenum.

Wheaton, B. (1997). The nature of chronic stress. In B. Gottlieb (Ed.), *Coping with chronic stress* (pp. 43–73). New York: Plenum.

Wheaton, B., & Clarke, P. (2003). Space meets time: Integrating temporal and contextual influences on mental health in early adulthood. *American Sociological Review*, *68*, 680–706.

Wheaton, B., Young, M., Montazer, S., & Stuart-Lahman, K. (2013). Social stress in the twenty-first century. In C. Aneshensel, J. Phelan, & A. Bierman (Eds.), *Handbook of the sociology of mental health* (pp. 299–323). New York: Springer.

Whitehead, K. (2022). How covid-19 quarantine isolation in Hong Kong is hurting mental health amid reports of suicide attempts at Penny's Bay; experts offer tips on managing feelings. *The South China Morning Post*. Retrieved from www.scmp.com/lifestyle/health-wellness/article/3168650/how-covid-19-quarantine-isolation-hong-kong-hurting

Williams, D., & Collins, C. (2001). Racial residential segregation: A fundamental cause of racial disparities in health. *Public Health Reports*, *116*, 404–416.

Zannas, A. S., & Chrousos, G. P. (2017). Epigenetic programming by stress and glucocorticoids along the human lifespan. *Molecular Psychiatry*, *22*(5), 640–646.

2 Cultural Beliefs About Mental Health

Gender Ideology, Emotional Suppression, and the Stigmatization of Mental Health

The Significance of Culture

Culture is an underappreciated force and analytical lens with which to examine the issue of mental health in East Asia. To illustrate, previous studies have found that East Asians typically are more reluctant to seek services for the treatment of distress compared to other groups (Tiwari & Wang, 2008). According to the U.S. Department of Health and Human Services (2001), this is true even of East Asians who immigrate to America, where only a small proportion of Asian Americans who are very likely to have a mental disorder, fulfilling the criteria for a diagnosis in the Diagnostic and Statistical Manual of Mental Disorders, seek services (Akutsu & Chu, 2006). Abe-Kim et al.'s (2007) study using a national sample of Asian Americans, which included a broad variety of mental health disorders among both foreign and U.S.-born Asian Americans, identified lower rates of mental health service use among Asian Americans (8.6% of the total sample sought mental health-related services).

The neglect of mental health and culture in East Asia is compounded by a neglect of the subject in sociological studies of mental health, little of which has been written about Asians. This is not to imply a lack of sociological research on the mental health of minorities and immigrants but rather a lack of attention devoted to this area in terms of fundamental elements of East Asian culture (Kramer et al., 2002). This clearly evokes a disconnection between our (academic and popular) understanding of mental health and grassroots experiences of mental health.

This chapter examines the familial ideals and norms of East Asian cultures, grounded on Confucianist principles, as they influence and/or are relevant to the mental health of families who belong to such cultures. This chapter does not attempt to generalize these cultures and dismiss their histories and geographies, nor does it suggest they are reducible to any one or more traits discussed here. Rather, this chapter schematically unpacks the cultural principles at work in East Asian cultures, and their intersection with mental health through their impact on coping resources, everyday life, and common deleterious mental health consequences.

DOI:10.4324/9781003308720-2

The Architecture of East Asian Culture: Stigma, Ideology, and Mental Health

There are cultural differences between China, Japan, and South Korea. Such differences surface in management and communication styles (Silverthorne, 2004). Japanese organizations, for instance, tend to motivate their networks by simulating *kaizen* – the idea that every employee and manager is a member of the same family, a management style intended to erase social boundaries, encourage open communication between workers and management, and incentivize productivity (Brunet & New, 2003). Chinese culture, by contrast, tends instead to preserve social boundaries and restrict information flow instead to enact a kind of particularistic trust (Bian, 2018, 2019).

Despite these differences, however, there are commonalities that cultures in China, Japan, and South Korea share – a set of values that they boil down to in their DNA as East Asian cultures. Above all, East Asian cultures are oriented toward communitarianism. This consists of placing the needs of a larger social unit above one's own, most of all the family, though also friend circles and colleagues. The way one comes to evaluate themselves, therefore, is entirely bound up in the contribution and service one provides to the larger groups that they belong to (Lee, 1985).

The primordial social unit, the North Star, that all the rules of East Asian cultures point to is the family. Policies that include mental health are thus shaped by this emphasis on the family, affording them disproportionate powers over individual treatment. Individuals can be involuntarily admitted if their families consent them to admission in East Asia. This practice is legalized in Japan and South Korea. It is not yet legalized in China, but still permitted provided there is family consent. Moreover, the Chinese system permits even public officers to exercise involuntary admission.

East Asian cultures thus exact both beneficial and deleterious influences on mental health in terms of stress. Since East Asian cultures are highly collectivistic, people's autonomy and sense of control erode, creating stress. It further gives rise to behaviors that further compromise this autonomy, such as committing acts for the family rather than for the self per obligations to the family – to maintain a sense of filial piety. It renders the individual more susceptible to indoctrination by family traditions, such as the discouragement of mental health treatment for social status.

Mental health, however, is poorly understood in East Asia. Part of this owes to the modern history of East Asian development which, for the most part, has been a story of survival. For most of the twentieth century, China, Korea, and Japan reeled from aftershocks of the Second World War. Korea was struck by internal strife that peaked in the Korean war and decades of authoritarian rule afterward. China experimented with lackluster economic policies that strove to move the nation from agrarian to modern modes of production. While Japan was comparatively better off than China and Korea, its economy notoriously tumbled in the 1980s with the collapse of its real estate and asset bubble.

The economic pressures throughout this long process of modernization primed inhabitants of the region toward physical survival. As such, there was historically little consciousness about mental health, despite the rise of mental health disorders during this period of instability. This specter of indifference lingers on today. People in the region do not understand what mental health is, which is why they don't value it in the first place. And it's *because* they don't value it that attritional coping resources for mental health are dismissed and problems go unchecked until they've evolved to extremes.

This is the basis of one family tradition that stifles mental health in East Asia. *Mental illness is traditionally defined as a curse inflicted on families, rather than a legitimate disorder*. Depression and its causes, for instance, are believed to be a natural part of life (Bernstein, 2007), while other mental health disorders are dismissed unfortunate predicaments for which no remedy exists. East Asians appear to only seek professional help if a mental illness has progressed to the manifestation of psychotic or dangerous behaviors, instead of in their preliminary stages where they are more easily curbed, such as personal problems or emotional distress (Yang et al., 2008).

Similarly, *it is believed in East Asian cultures that maturity is the ability to control personal feelings, particularly those of discontent*. Given that self-esteem comes from helping the family in communitarian East Asian cultures, avoidance of confrontation is valorized. As a result, emotional turmoil is naturalized as a part of life, toward which a responsible and mature adult would contain this psychologically by repressing their emotions. This has given rise to a common hesitation among East Asians toward broaching the subject of emotions or discussing reflections (Kim et al., 2002). Furthermore, they are generally encouraged to communicate more through nonverbal or metaphorical means (Uba, 1994).

Another preeminent value in East Asian cultures that arises is *social status, commonly referred to as face.*

Cultural sociologists observe the significance of social status as a symbolic means of building distinctions between individuals (Lamont & Fournier, 1992; Clair et al., 2016). It allows people on a basic level to socially differentiate individuals in terms of their work and achievements. It can be a source of striving, as people look to these differentiations as a guidepost for their own professional and life decisions, pursuing a better job. More often, however, these differentiations enact a kind of social distance between actors. Social distance does not mean physical distance, as is ubiquitously conceived of in an age of COVID-19, but rather the refusal to connect with or ostracization of someone. Pierre Bourdieu aptly called this symbolic violence (Bourdieu & Wacquant,

1992, pp. 167–168) or discrimination by actors assigned to higher statuses against those with lower statuses, such that the cultural meanings behind their status differences reinforce their inequality.

My research on medical organizations and professional firms in East Asia shows that higher statuses are assigned greater moral worth, which leads to more opportunities. The actors within these social spaces who have the most status are blessed with the most opportunities for financial profit, collaborations, information exchange, and success overall. In a year-long ethnography of cosmetic surgery clinics in South Korea, for instance, I observed that patients who have had cosmetic surgery are perceived by peers, colleagues, and friends to have a higher status (Au, 2022a, 2022b). Across all kinds of professions, people who decided to undergo cosmetic surgery subsequently had the benefit of connecting with higher-ups in their workplaces and more invitations to social activities.

Similar patterns emerged in financial and legal firms in the region. Tracing the amounts of financial technology that flowed through financial firms, I found that firms and banks with the greatest amounts of financial technology were the most likely to have connections with other firms in the region (Au, 2022c). Using network analyses of law firm partner moves in Hong Kong over the past 20 years, I also observed that those firms with the highest status attracted the most talent (Liu & Au, 2019; Liu et al., 2022). Put differently, the winners took all. The structural symmetry of these social distances and status structures – that status begets more status – across these different organizational forms and contexts speaks to the rigidity and sway of the beliefs in East Asian cultures.

Status or face matters tremendously in East Asian cultures because status is not merely individual for the East Asian resident beholden to the honor of their larger social unit; status is also communal in nature. Individual status reflects on their families, their friends, and close contacts. This is exacerbated by the fact that East Asian networks are especially dense and interconnected, as will be shown in Chapter 3. Actors are therefore significantly embedded in their group memberships and social units, and the cultural beliefs underpinning their interactions – like the moral worth assigned to face – are especially difficult to budge. The rich social embeddedness that characterizes East Asian networks is thus relatively impervious to change, at the same time it facilitates the diffusion of information through their networks quicker. Status is also something that gets transmitted quickly.

Part of why opportunities are herded to those with high status owes to such East Asian network arrangements and cultural beliefs that characterize face as something contagious and communal. People are more willing to associate with high-status friends, hoping that their star power might rub off on them. In East Asian cultures that emphasize reciprocity between actors within the same network, it pays even more to network with and help out high-status friends, motivated by the belief that they could owe you a favor and repay it for tasks that you might be excluded from because of your status, such as job information about an internal posting in a company.

Coupled with the traditional Confucian emphasis on the importance of family above individual needs, people are driven by the pressure to elevate their family's social status. Seeking treatment for – and even acknowledging mental health problems – may be conceived as smearing the family honor with shame (Bernstein, 2007), therefore impeding emotional acceptance of one's stresses and the search for solutions.

This manifests in various ways to suppress different identities within the family. Mental health can be further considered in the context of separate generations (Huang et al., 2012). For children, educational competition and academic stress are among the greatest stressors. Since education is widely regarded as a way to move up within familial traditions, children are pushed to pursue superior academic performances, which also reflect on their families. As a result, children are faced with immense pressure to perform and intense stigma if they fail to obtain educational merit and especially those who engage in delinquency.

Huang et al. (2012) discovered that children's exclusive dedication to education made them less likely to develop externalizing problems and had higher self-control. Studies have also found that East Asian children may be less inclined to behave problematically or in delinquent ways that could compromise family status, they also exhibit greater rates of clinically impairing internalizing problems, namely depression, social anxiety, and suicide (Austin & Chorpita, 2004; Choi et al., 2006; Lee et al., 2001; Okazaki, 2000). Thus, this dedication to academics and familial status creates stressors that may be too difficult for social support to adequately buffer.

Rigorous expectations of education create social isolation among East Asian children. These practices precipitate into poorer quality of social life, effectively depreciating their potential to develop social networks that could alleviate the immense stress they commonly experience. When children are deprived of interpersonal skills, they become socially inept and thus culturally isolated.

Similarly, for social status, adults are obliged to disregard mental health disorders, avoid professional mental health treatment, dedicate themselves to the future of their families, and persist in their assigned roles: children as students, men as breadwinners, women as submissive supports (Bernstein, 2007). For women, there also exists a sexism that dominates East Asian familial structures, organizing it around a patriarchal system in which females are expected to be complacent and supportive. For example, mothers are pressured to replicate the image of a submissive wife and a sacrificial mother (Chang & Kim, 1988; Fan & Qian, 2022). Consequently, mothers may be encouraged to take on more household duties and may even experience marital distress when they step outside the housewife ideal, such as by contributing to household earnings (Furdyna et al., 2008). All these pressures add up to give fuel to mental health disorders such as depression and anxiety, at the same time sap individuals of interpersonal skills, self-esteem, and sense of control.

Coping Resources and Mental Health Problems in East Asia

East Asian cultures do lend some unique tools for individuals to cope with stress. Some of these resources include social support, which shields individuals from mental health problems in East Asian populations (De La Rosa & White, 2001; Prati & Pietrantoni, 2010). These protective effects are further documented in intervention studies with East Asians (Dobkin et al., 2002; Thompson et al., 2001). This is especially the case considering the collectivistic orientation and emphasis on belonging to a larger social unit that serves as the bedrock of East Asian cultures.

In some studies of the mental health of Asian immigrant workers, the suggested buffering effects of social support on social discrimination, job and employment concerns for the immigrant, or mental health problems and substance use are unobserved (Tsai & Thompson, 2013). Emotional support from family or friends may mitigate stress and prevent the emergence of adverse mental health or substance use problems, but this effect may be leavened for serious stressors like social discrimination.

Social support primarily comes from family or ethnic communities, providing a supportive environment for the second generation (Portes & Rumbaut, 2001) as well as emotional support for coping with external challenges in acculturation (Wierzbicki, 2004; Wong & Mock, 1997).

Mastery, the individual perception of ability to handle stress (Salas et al., 2013), would likely be low for the immigrant. The higher one's socioeconomic status is, the higher his/her educational and occupational prospect, leading to reassurance of secure futures and higher self-confidence (Schieman & Plickert, 2008). Given the typical immigrant's immense debts and low socioeconomic status (Huang et al., 2012), self-esteem may be volatile. Inability to communicate with sufficient language proficiency and unawareness of the host country's culture, norms, and systems could additionally depreciate one's sense of control and self-confidence.

Emotional suppression becomes a common coping resource for Asian immigrants per cultural traditions (Pang, 1990). A stark cross-cultural distinction exists between Asian values and Western values in the function of emotional suppression: in a study of Americans of different ethnicities, emotional suppression was found less harmful in Asian Americans, in contrast to the deleterious effects observed with others with Western European values (Butler et al., 2007). We can thus infer that emotional suppression is a function of Asian values (mark of maturity) and may serve as a kind of social resource, other cultures.

However, emotional suppression also comes with negative consequences, including avoidance, reluctance to share emotions, reduced social support, less relationship closeness, and less social likability (Butler et al., 2003; Gross, 2002; Gross & John, 2003; John & Gross, 2004). As very little research exists on suppression (Butler et al., 2007), the extent of this effect should be explored in the context of Asian immigrants, rather than native-born Asian Americans. More focus should thus be attributed to recognizing discrepancies between collectivistic and individualistic cultures, as well as acculturated and recently adapting immigrant, to develop a holistic framework through which mental health issues and the mediating influence of culture are better understood.

This is true of civilians and celebrities alike.

On a cold evening in 2017, when the sun began to desert the sky, a cornerstone of the burgeoning Korean pop (K-pop) industry left into the gathering dark. Jong-hyun was the lead singer of SHINee and the face of K-pop's global influence at the peak of its popularity. His body was found in a rented apartment in Gangnam-gu, an affluent district widely synonymous with luxury and wealth in South Korea. The cause of death was determined to be suicide. In a farewell note he left, he wrote,

> I am broken from inside. The depression that had been slowly eating me up finally devoured me and I couldn't defeat it.
>
> (Wang, 2017)

More than idols, SHINee was an icon of an industry, bringing newfound attention to a country we had scarcely heard of but would valorize for years to come. Over the past decade since their inception, the industry has swollen to become a powerful machine, churning out idols from a mold.

From the sandstorm unsettled by Jong-hyun's death, there exist deep problems marking the shadow of his legacy; problems that his death has proved to be perennial concerning celebrity culture itself in the K-pop industry. Hankyung's famous departure from SuperJunior in 2009 tabled challenges of fame that prominent K-pop idols have evoked since, from fellow band member Lee Eunhyuk to Jong-hyun.

Headlines blared once more in 2019 when Goo Hara and Sulli passed away – both for suspected suicide (Choe & Lee, 2019). Pressures from talent management and entertainment companies bent on rendering individuals into stars by supplanting flesh with steel, man with machine in a stirring engine for profit. Faustian contracts that bind stars to micromanaged schedules, freedoms, activities, and successes. Risk of abuse from powerful figures in companies who hold the reins on their careers. Already isolated from the normalcy of a settled life, they are surrounded by an ocean of blind, waving, screaming fans. Unable to be taken seriously when they express their problems, they are doubly bound in silence by the taboo of mental health, whose problems are forbidden from acknowledgment. They are often denied and dismissed as natural symptoms of stress, expected to go away with age and maturity. And even when they do not, we blindly hold on to the opposite, trusting the glow from the stars would shield them from the cold of space, trusting in the certainty of tomorrow like acolytes to an altar. But by the time we realize this isn't the case, it already becomes too late.

"If anyone knew what being famous was really about," Sia once recalled in a 2013 interview, "no one would want fame. . . . [I]t is a monster that questions everything there is to question. Even things I had never thought to question. Things I had never dreamed of feeling insecure about." As a tribute to her growing concerns about privacy, she boldly created her trademark: an oversized bob-cut wig to mask all the parts of her face that we would recognize her with, but wouldn't. Although it typically evokes much fanfare and excitement from fans worldwide, there is much more significant to the act than we think.

Interviews I conducted with youth on the subject of mental health confirm the health benefits of privacy, as something just as important as social support. They report that privacy offers a space where one can simply exist freely, be however they wish, do whatever they wish, and live bereft of judgment, if not obligation, to the social demands that the rest of life imposes. Privacy affords a human sense of freedom that pop stars are forbidden to breathe.

Jong-hyun passed like a whisper and, in a sense of remorseful irony, that was the only shred of privacy he had ever had. Where Sia carved out a space for freedom and privacy in the anonymity of a wig, Jong-hyun sought it out in the next world, since he couldn't find it in this one. Faced with lack of privacy, stars are torn from the arms of security and cast out into the night sky – to glow for fans who fail to notice the sea of blackness that surrounds them; that stars hang in the sky by dangling on invisible ropes that crawl towards their necks.

A cultural approach thus offers a useful analytical framework with which to identify the sources and experience of stress as rooted in cultural beliefs that may even transcend, though not erase, social classes. Jong-hyun's, Goo Hara's, and Sulli's deaths are tragic blips in a growing cluster of mental health illnesses on the climb in East Asia. Their deaths show that this is not about the K-pop idol profession. This is about a public health issue of grave significance. A study published in 2018 in *BMC Psychiatry* (Jang et al., 2018), a leading journal in psychiatry, analyzed data from a nationally representative survey in South Korea to tell a grim story about mental health. Only 16% of people with depressive symptoms, including suicidality, actually seek out mental health consultation. Formal, professional help is also discouraged in light of the cultural stigma associated with even the recognition of mental health disorders, perceived as curses to the family, and the cultural perception that equates maturity with emotional suppression (Kim et al., 2002). As a result, professional mental health services and treatment are deprived of the same resources and respect as general health services.

For stars and for ordinary civilians alike, the chains of East Asian cultures may shake themselves into a noose. Everyone needs a village, even stars who flicker out into the wind – broken souls that public opinion is too busy worshipping to try to understand, to mend, to see the ironic powerlessness in a position of privilege. Among traditional East Asian norms that valorize apathy as a sign of strength and malign feeling as unproductive and weak, individuals lose a fundamental part of the human condition: emotion. Banished from our being, there exists little room for addressing distress and mental health.

From One Culture to Another

What happens when people migrate? Although strong connection to a tight ethnic community is identified as a catalyst for assimilation (Portes & Rumbaut, 2001), there may be cultural drawbacks. The impact of stressors and the buffer effects of coping resources is much more variable for migrants (Agudelo-Suárez et al., 2009; Noh & Kaspar, 2003; Tsai & Thompson, 2013), but one thing that continues to hold steadfast is the set of ideologies and values that scaffold East Asian cultures, creating opportunities and problems for individuals and families.

Migration typically creates financial precarity for families, which naturally brings up stressors to do with subsistence, lack of recreation, and ability to afford social services (Huang et al., 2012). Stressors may also arise in everyday life when immigrants are required to adapt to new languages, which facilitates how well a person is adapting or acculturating to a new culture. Among East Asian American immigrants, those with less proficiency in English perceive greater mental health needs than those with more proficiency (Nguyen, 2011). People who are less fluent are more likely to be socially isolated, less interactive, and have access to fewer relationships – straining their personal coping resources even further.

However, for East Asian individuals, there is additional distress when they become immersed in a new culture. East Asian cultures have been found to be more resistant to change and challenge than even other cultures in the Asia-Pacific region – which leads to cultural clashes that create tensions within families (Choi & Thomas, 2009).

Tightknit families like those in East Asian cultures may prevent members from adopting new norms to displace traditional ones (Feliciano, 2001; Gibson, 2001; Zhou, 2004). In lieu of submission, for example, women may be exposed to and encouraged toward accepting the idea of a more autonomous mother. Kim (1985) notes that this creates a new social reality built on biculturalism: a mother's mentality is shaped by her social environment that bifurcates into the East Asian traditional community and the American majority society. Failure to adapt to this new sociocultural setting could be a chronic stressor for her, possibly creating a sense of helplessness, misplacement, and loss of identity.

The erosion of the submissive wife ideal becomes a traumatic stressor for her family. While her autonomy allows for fewer emotional problems within her person, problems emerge in her family: she could obtain autonomy in manners perceived nonchalant or even hostile by her family. For example, socializing with friends more than fulfilling domestic roles at home, resulting in an immoderate balance between family and social life. Deviation from the ideal could cause distress for the other members from shock, leading to disagreements between, and emotional problems for, both parties, unable to cope. Indeed, a recent psychological study of Asian American women shows that immigrants often experience less familial support and greater stress overall (Morey et al., 2020).

Thus, adapting to cultures outside of East Asian cultures can constitute a momentous determinant of mental health. Choi and Thomas (2009) contend that attitudes toward adaptation itself are affected by education and English fluency, in addition to cultural organization and values. Their study revealed that East Asians were the most resistant to acculturation.

Within East Asian cultures, the rigidity of these expectations for how families are structured may worsen the stress of migration and cultural changes. To illustrate, immigrants typically suffer losses in social support due to the physical displacement from these networks in their home country and receive fewer opportunities to build new connections in host countries on account of language, cultural, and socioeconomic status barriers (Pearlin & Bierman, 2013). This cutoff from sources of support outside the family may pose unique dangers to the mental health of East Asian individuals, who have little recourse but to rely on their families – the same families that culturally mandate emotional suppression and consider stress to be a matter of maturity, rather than mental health.

In the Wake of Emotional Suppression: Substance Abuse in East Asia

Drug and alcohol abuse are recurrent problems in East Asia. Figure 2.1 shows cases of drug and alcohol abuse in 100,000 people in East Asia. Disaggregating the results by country, China, Japan, and South Korea, shows little difference. Substance abuse continues to be a serious problem in all three countries.

There are several cultural reasons for this. First, the *collectivistic push of East Asian cultures* may foster the desire to fit in: to appease the cultural goal of social harmony in a group through shared practices. Thus, an individual may not perceive his/her practices as harmful not simply due to peer pressure, but for the support he/she is giving to the group

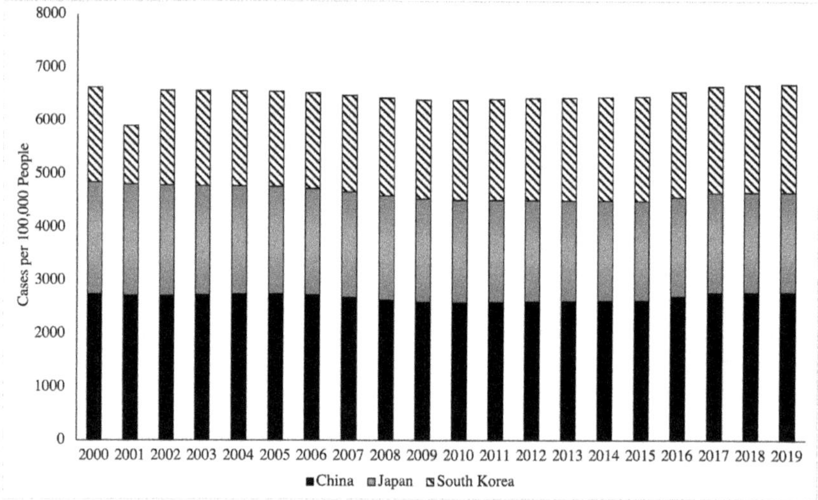

Figure 2.1 Cases of drug and alcohol abuse in 100,000 people in East Asia (2000–2019).

Source: Author's calculations using data from the Global Burden of Disease Collaborative Network (2020)

by promoting a practice they can all partake in to foster solidarity. East Asian cultures also encourage heavy drinking during social occasions, especially among adult males (Lim & Chang, 2009).

Second, the *patriarchy* that is part of traditional East Asian cultures. In a systematic review of alcohol use disorders in China, a review of all major research studies published on the subject, Cheng and colleagues (2015) at the Shanghai Jiao Tong University comprehensively find that the current prevalence of dependence on alcohol disorders is about 2.2% and lifetime dependence jumps to 3.7% – levels that rival the United States and Australia. What's striking about this alcoholism, they find, is that it mostly occurs among men. This picture is corroborated in Japan and South Korea by scholars who identify men as the most likely to be binge drinkers and abuse alcohol consumption compared to women (Choe et al., 2018; Sugaya et al., 2021).

Third, substance abuse may be popular as a way to fill the void left by the cultural *demand to suppress emotions*, particularly in face of life adversity. When East Asians are deprived of social support and their personal coping resources wane in potency, they may feel the need to resort to alcohol or substance use to alleviate stress, especially when communicating about feelings is construed as immature.

The COVID-19 pandemic has now exacerbated everyday adversities for households and invited unprecedented levels of stress in East Asia

(Ryu et al., 2021). In a telling, large-scale study of the impact of COVID-19 in Japan, Sugaya and colleagues (2021) identify a new battery of challenges that ordinary households have been subject to. Families struggled to pay bills, lost jobs and income, experienced difficulty procuring COVID-19 protections (e.g., masks), and had their working and school schedules drastically disrupted – on top of anxieties from the health risks of contracting the virus itself. What resulted was a surge of depression and anxiety – and alcohol abuse to cope with the myriad stressors they faced. Moreover, the researchers found that people's sources of social support and connections to others outside the family were fewer than before the pandemic. Likewise, Tchimtchoua Tamo (2020) observed that mothers in China experience greater isolation and distress than before the pandemic, owing to a combination of economic pressures and struggles with caring for their families without adequate child support. Sun and colleagues (2020) extend this to demonstrate increased substance abuse behaviors during the pandemic in China, particularly alcohol, tobacco, and new addictions like internet use.

As bad as substance abuse problems may be, they have a long history in East Asian populations in no small part because of their cultural ideologies and stigma of mental health (Chi et al., 1989; Choi, 1997; Legge & Sherlock, 1991; Yamamoto et al., 1994). The problem continues to grow when we realize that mental health problems rooted in stress do not stay idle. Like a fire spreading atop crossed circuits, drug and alcohol abuse tend to lead to other health problems both directly and indirectly. The direct problems are better documented, such as liver disease and cancer (Meyerhoff et al., 2005). Indirect problems, however, are far more social and less understood, such as partner violence.

Research on domestic violence in East Asia is limited and nascent, but the problem remains very much a real and urgent issue. Statistical analyses of national data in Korea found that domestic violence stood at 16.5% in 2010 and 12.1% in 2016, the latest figures. More concerning, however, is that the overwhelming majority of this violence was perpetrated by men *against women* (Han & Choi, 2021; Kim et al., 2016). This is much the same in China. Though data on the prevalence of domestic violence nationwide are not available in China, city-wide surveys have identified gender roles as a primary driver of dating violence against women (Ren & Zhang, 2018; Zhang & Zhao, 2018). Japan reports low amounts of partner violence, about 1.1% in the general population (Kageyama et al., 2018). However, among the cases of violence that occur, gender relations and ideologies – about what the place of a woman is in relation to a man – play a pivotal role (Shire & Nemoto, 2020).

In addition to the gendered pattern of domestic violence, evidence shows that this violence is accentuated among men of lower class and who have lower levels of education (Kim et al., 2016). Domestic violence patterns reflect the patriarchal familial structure that favors the husband's position over the wife's, making the wife the common victim of abuse (Han et al., 2010). Even for migrants, husbands who abuse alcohol, coupled with diminished social support and personal coping resources, are more prone to act violently toward their wives (Han et al., 2010).

This is a useful heuristic with which to end this chapter. How are stressors – and stress itself – perceived by members of East Asian, collectivistic cultures? While families in Asian cultures can bolster ability to cope with stress by acting as a form of social support, their patriarchal ideology, collectivistic concern about status, and suppression of emotions exert a chilling effect on experiences of mental health in families. Despite much evidence of mental health issues in East Asia, stigmatization of mental health as a curse to the family continues to persist.

Put simply, men who face hardships and naturally experience distress are left unable to cope by cultures that tell them emotional hardships are a mere matter of maturity. As a result, men are forced to find ways to vent their frustrations, resulting in the dual poisons of substance abuse and domestic violence. This abuse then increases depression and decreases mastery and self-esteem not only in women but in their children as well. Victims are similarly driven by cultural norms to suppress pent-up stress from abuse and refuse to resist it from patriarchal abusers (Rhodes & McKenzie, 1998). These groups consequently become more susceptible to depression, posttraumatic stress, and issues with social or interpersonal functioning (Gordon, 2000; Lee, 2003).

As this chapter has demonstrated, perceptions of mental health derived from culture must be accounted for and addressed in treatment settings to improve access to professional help. The rest of this book attempts to do just that.

References

Abe-Kim, J., Takeuchi, D. T., Hong, S., Zane, N., Sue, S., Spencer, M. S., Appel, H., Nicdao, E., & Alegria, M. (2007). Use of mental health – Related services among immigrant and US-born Asian Americans: Results from the National Latino and Asian American study. *American Journal of Public Health*, *97*(1), 91–98.

Agudelo-Suárez, A., Gil-Gonzalez, D., Ronda-Perez, E., Porthe, V., Paramio-Perez, G., Garcia, A. M., & Gari, A. (2009). Discrimination, work and health in immigrant populations in Spain. *Journal of Social Science and Medicine*, *68*, 1866–1874.

Akutsu, P., & Chu, J. (2006). Clinical problems that initiate professional help seeking behaviors from Asian Americans. *Professional Psychology: Research and Practice*, *37*, 407–415.

Au, A. (2022a). An ethnographic toolkit for studying networking pathways of hard-to-reach populations: The case of cosmetic surgery consumers in South Korea. *International Journal of Qualitative Methods*, 21 (Online First). DOI: 10.1177/16094069221101962.

Au, A. (2022b). Transnational cross-cultural research: Modern challenges and solutions for field access, data collection, and analysis. In P. Liamputtong (Ed.), *Handbook of qualitative cross-cultural research* (pp. 335–355). Cheltenham: Edward Elgar.

Au, A. (2022c). FinTech innovation and knowledge flows in Hong Kong's financial sector: A social network analysis approach. *Journal of Asia Business Studies*, *16*(2), 294–307.

Austin, A. A., & Chorpita, B. F. (2004). Temperament, anxiety, and depression: Comparisons across five ethnic groups of children. *Journal of Clinical Child and Adolescent Psychology*, *33*, 216–226.

Bernstein, K. S. (2007). Mental health issues among urban Korean American immigrants. *Journal of Transcultural Nursing*, *18*, 175–180.

Bian, Y. (2018). The prevalence and the increasing significance of Guanxi. *The China Quarterly*, *235*(3), 597–621.

Bian, Y. (2019). *Guanxi, how China works*. New York: John Wiley & Sons.

Bourdieu, P., & Wacquant, L. (1992). *An invitation to reflexive sociology*. Chicago, IL: University of Chicago Press.

Brunet, A. P., & New, S. (2003). Kaizen in Japan: An empirical study. *International Journal of Operations & Production Management*, *23*(12), 1426–1446.

Butler, E. A., Egloff, B., Wilhelm, F. H., Smith, N. C., Erickson, E. A., & Gross, J. J. (2003). The social consequences of expressive suppression. *Emotion*, *3*, 48–67.

Butler, E. A., Lee, T. L., & Gross, J. J. (2007). Emotion regulation and culture: Are the social consequences of emotion suppression culture-specific? *Emotion*, *7*(1), 30–48.

Chang, H. J., & Kim, H. W. (1988). The study of the "house-wife syndrome" in Korea – with special concern with neurotic symptoms and family strains. *Asian Family Mental Health Conference Proceedings*. Psychiatric Research Institute of Tokyo, Tokyo.

Cheng, H. G., Deng, F., Xiong, W., & Phillips, M. R. (2015). Prevalence of alcohol use disorders in mainland China: A systematic review. *Addiction*, *110*(5), 761–774.

Chi, I., Lubben, J., & Kitano, H. (1989). Differences in drinking behavior among three Asian American groups. *Journal of Studies on Alcohol*, *50*, 15–23.

Choe, S., & Lee, S. (2019). Suicides by K-pop stars prompt soul-searching in South Korea. *The New York Times*. Retrieved from https://www.nytimes.com/2019/11/25/world/asia/goo-hara-kpop-suicide.html

Choe, S. A., Yoo, S., JeKarl, J., & Kim, K. K. (2018). Recent trend and associated factors of harmful alcohol use based on age and gender in Korea. *Journal of Korean Medical Science*, *33*(4).

Choi, G. (1997). Acculturation stress, social support, and depression in Korean American families. *Journal of Family Social Work*, *2*(1), 81–97.

Choi, H., Meininger, J. C., & Roberts, R. E. (2006). Ethnic differences in adolescents' mental distress, social stress, and resources. *Adolescence*, *41*, 263–283.

Choi, J. B., & Thomas, M. (2009) Predictive factors of acculturation attitudes and social support among Asian immigrants in the USA. *International Journal of Social Welfare*, *18*, 76–84.

Clair, M., Daniel, C., & Lamont, M. (2016). Destigmatization and health: Cultural constructions and the long-term reduction of stigma. *Social Science & Medicine*, *165*, 223–232.

De La Rosa, M. R., & White, M. S. (2001). A review of the role of social support systems in the drug use behavior of Hispanics. *Journal of Psychoactive Drugs*, *33*, 233–240.

Dobkin, P. L., Civita, M. D., Paraherakis, A., & Gill, K. (2002). The role of functional social support in treatment retention and outcomes among outpatient adult substance abusers. *Addiction*, *97*, 347–356.

Fan, W., & Qian, Y. (2022). Constellations of gender ideology, earnings arrangements, and marital satisfaction: A comparison across four East Asian societies. *Asian Population Studies*, *18*(1), 24–40.

Feliciano, C. (2001). The benefits of biculturalism: Exposure to immigrant culture and dropping out of school among Asian and Latino youths. *Social Science Quarterly*, *82*, 865–879.

Furdyna, H. E., Tucker, M. B., & James, A. D. (2008). Relative spousal earnings and marital happiness among African American and white women. *Journal of Marriage and Family*, *70*(2), 332–344.

Gibson, M. A. (2001). Immigrant adaptation and patterns of acculturation. *Human Development*, *44*, 19–23.

Gordon, M. (2000). Definitional issues in violence against women. *Violence against Women*, *6*, 747–783.

Gross, J. J. (2002). Emotion regulation: Affective, cognitive, and social consequences. *Psychophysiology*, *39*, 281–291.

Gross, J. J., & John, O. P. (2003). Individual differences in two emotion regulation processes: Implications for affect, relationships, and well-being. *Journal of Personality and Social Psychology*, *85*, 348–362.

Han, A. D., Kim, E. J., & Tyson, S. Y. (2010). Partner violence against Korean immigrant women. *Journal of Transcultural Nursing*, *21*, 370–376.

Han, Y. R., & Choi, H. Y. (2021). Risk factors affecting intimate partner violence occurrence in South Korea: Findings from the 2016 domestic violence survey. *PLoS One*, *16*(3), e0247916.

Huang, K.-Y., Calzada, E., Cheng, S., & Brotman, L. M. (2012). Physical and mental health disparities among young children of Asian immigrants. *Journal of Pediatrics*, *160*, 331–336.

Jang, J., Lee, S. A., Kim, W., Choi, Y., & Park, E. C. (2018). Factors associated with mental health consultation in South Korea. *BMC Psychiatry*, *18*(1), 17–28.

John, O. P., & Gross, J. J. (2004). Healthy and unhealthy emotion regulation: Personality processes, individual differences, and life span development. *Journal of Personality*, *72*, 1301–1333.

Kageyama, M., Solomon, P., Yokoyama, K., Nakamura, Y., Kobayashi, S., & Fujii, C. (2018). Violence towards family caregivers by their relative with schizophrenia in Japan. *Psychiatric Quarterly*, *89*(2), 329–340.

Kim, B. (1985). The social reality of the Korean-American women: Toward crashing with the Confucian ideology. In I. S. Lee (Ed.), *Korean American women: Toward self-realization* (pp. 65–97). Mansfield, OH: Han Geul Printing Co.

Kim, J. Y., Oh, S., & Nam, S. I. (2016). Prevalence and trends in domestic violence in South Korea: Findings from national surveys. *Journal of Interpersonal Violence*, *31*(8), 1554–1576.

Kim, M. J., Cho, H., Cheon-Klessig, Y., Gerace, L., & Camilleri, D. (2002). Primary health care for Korean immigrants: Sustaining a culturally sensitive model. *Public Health Nursing*, *19*, 191–200.

Kramer, E. J., Kwong, K., Lee, E., & Chung, H. (2002). Cultural factors influencing the mental health of Asian Americans. *Western Journal of Medicine*, *176*, 227–231.

Lamont, M., & Fournier, M. (Eds.). (1992). *Cultivating differences: Symbolic boundaries and the making of inequality*. Chicago, IL: University of Chicago Press.

Lee, I. S. (Ed.). (1985). *Korean American women: Toward self-realization*. Mansfield, OH: Han Geul Printing Co.

Lee, J., Lei, A., & Sue, S. (2001). The current state of mental health research on Asian Americans. *Journal of Human Behavior in the Social Environment*, *3*, 159–178.

Lee, S. B. (2003). Working with Korean-American families: Multicultural hermeneutics in understanding and dealing with marital domestic violence. *American Journal of Family Therapy*, *31*, 159–178.

Legge, C., & Sherlock, L. (1991). Perception of alcohol use and misuse in three ethnic communities: Implications for prevention programming. *The International Journal of the Addictions*, *25*, 629–653.

Lim, L. L., & Chang, W. C. (2009). Role of collective self-esteem on youth violence in a collective culture. *International Journal of Psychology*, *44*, 71–78.

Liu, S., & Au, A. (2019). The gateway to global China: Hong Kong and the future of Chinese law firms. *Wisconsin International Law Journal*, *37*, 308–349.

Liu, S., Blocq, D., Honari, A., & Au, A. (2022). Professional flows: Lateral moves of law firm partners in Hong Kong, 1994–2018. *Journal of Professions and Organization*, *9*(1), 1–19.

Meyerhoff, D. J., Bode, C., Nixon, S. J., de Bruin, E. A., Bode, J. C., & Seitz, H. K. (2005). Health risks of chronic moderate and heavy alcohol consumption: How much is too much? *Journal of Alcohol Clinical and Experimental Research*, *29*, 1334–1340.

Morey, B. N., Gee, G. C., Shariff-Marco, S., Yang, J., Allen, L., & Gomez, S. L. (2020). Ethnic enclaves, discrimination, and stress among Asian American women: Differences by nativity and time in the United States. *Cultural Diversity and Ethnic Minority Psychology*, *26*(4), 460–471.

Nguyen, D. (2011). Acculturation and perceived mental health need among older Asian immigrants. *Journal of Behavioral Health Services & Research*, *38*(4), 526–532.

Noh, S., & Kaspar, V. (2003). Perceived discrimination and depression: Moderating effects of coping, acculturation, and ethnic support. *American Journal of Public Health*, *93*, 232–238.

Okazaki, S. (2000). Asian American and white American differences on affective distress symptoms: Do symptom reports differ across reporting methods? *Journal Cross Cultural Psychology*, *31*, 603–625.

Pang, K. Y. C. (1990). Hwabyung: The construction of a Korean popular illness among Korean elderly immigrant women in the United States. *Culture, Medicine, and Psychiatry*, *14*, 495–512.

Pearlin, L. I., & Bierman, A. (2013). Current issues and future directions in research into the stress process. In *Handbook of the sociology of mental health* (2nd ed.). New York: Springer. https://doi.org/10.1007/978-94-007-4276-5_16.

Portes, A., & Rumbaut, R. G. (2001). Conclusion. In R. Rumbaut & A. Portes (Eds.), *Ethnicities: Children of immigrants in America*. Los Angeles, CA: University of California Press.

Prati, G., & Pietrantoni, L. (2010). The relation of perceived and received social support to mental health among first responders: A meta-analytic review. *Journal Community Psychology*, *38*, 403–417.
Ren, L., & Zhang, H. (2018). Advancing empirical research on China's juvenile delinquency and juvenile justice: Continuity and expansion. *Journal of Contemporary Criminal Justice*, *34*, 120–127.
Rhodes, N. R., & McKenzie, E. B. (1998). Why do battered women stay? Three decades of research. *Aggression and Violent Behavior*, *3*, 391–406.
Ryu, S., Park, I. H., Kim, M., Lee, Y. R., Lee, J., Kim, H., . . . Kim, S. W. (2021). Network study of responses to unusualness and psychological stress during the COVID-19 outbreak in Korea. *PLoS One*, *16*(2), e0246894.
Salas, L. M., Ayón, C., & Gurrola, M. (2013). Estamos traumados: The effect of anti-immigrant sentiment and policies on the mental health of Mexican immigrant families. *Journal of Community Psychology*, *41*(8), 1005–1020.
Schieman, S., & Plickert, G. (2008). How knowledge is power: Education and the sense of control. *Social Forces*, *87*, 153–183.
Shire, K. A., & Nemoto, K. (2020). The origins and transformations of conservative gender regimes in Germany and Japan. *Social Politics: International Studies in Gender, State & Society*, *27*(3), 432–448.
Silverthorne, C. (2004). The impact of organizational culture and person-organization fit on organizational commitment and job satisfaction in Taiwan. *Leadership & Organization Development Journal*, *25*(7), 592–599.
Sugaya, N., Yamamoto, T., Suzuki, N., & Uchiumi, C. (2021). Alcohol use and its related psychosocial effects during the prolonged COVID-19 pandemic in Japan: A cross-sectional survey. *International Journal of Environmental Research and Public Health*, *18*(24), 13318–13334.
Sun, Y., Li, Y., Bao, Y., Meng, S., Sun, Y., Schumann, G., Kosten, T., Strang, J., Lu, L., & Shi, J. (2020). Brief report: Increased addictive internet and substance use behavior during the COVID-19 pandemic in China. *The American Journal on Addictions*, *29*(4), 268–270.
Tchimtchoua Tamo, A. R. (2020). An analysis of mother stress before and during COVID-19 pandemic: The case of China. *Health Care for Women International*, *41*(11–12), 1349–1362.
Thompson, E. A., Eggert, L. L., Randell, B. P., & Pike, K. C. (2001). Evaluation of indicated suicide risk prevention approaches for potential high school dropouts. *American Journal of Public Health*, *91*, 741–752.
Tiwari, S. K., & Wang, J. (2008). Ethnic differences in mental health service use among White, Chinese, South Asian and South East Asian populations living in Canada. *Social Psychiatry and Psychiatric Epidemiology*, *43*(11), 866–871.
Tsai, J. H.-C., & Thompson, E. A. (2013). Impact of social discrimination, job concerns, and social support on Filipino immigrant worker mental health and substance use. *American Journal of Industrial Medicine*, *56*, 1082–1094.
Uba, L. (1994). *Asian Americans: Personality patterns, identity, and mental health*. New York: Guilford.
U.S. Department of Health and Human Services. (2001). Mental health care for Asian Americans and Pacific Islanders. In *Mental health: Culture, race, and ethnicity a supplement to mental health: A report of the surgeon general* (pp. 107–126). Rockville, MD: U.S. Department of Health and Human

Services, Office of the Surgeon General, Substance Abuse and Mental Health Services Administration.

Wang, A. (2017, December 19). K-pop star's suicide note reveals pressures of fame, depression that 'consumed' him. *Washington Post*. Retrieved from www.washingtonpost.com/news/worldviews/wp/2017/12/19/k-pop-stars-suicide-note-reveals-depression-that-consumed-him-pressures-of-fame/

Wierzbicki, S. (2004). *Beyond the immigrant enclave*. New York: LFB Scholarly Publishing LLC.

Wong, L., & Mock, M. (1997). Asian American young adults. In E. Lee (Ed.), *Working with Asian American*. New York: The Guilford Press.

Yamamoto, J., Rhee, S., & Chang, D. (1994). Psychiatric disorders among elderly Koreans in the United States. *Community Mental Health Journal*, *30*(1), 17–27.

Yang, L. H., Phelan, J. C., & Link, B. G. (2008). Stigma towards traditional Chinese medicine and psychiatric treatment among Chinese-Americans. *Cultural Diversity and Ethnic Minority Psychology*, *14*, 10–18.

Zhang, H., & Zhao, R. (2018). Empirical research on domestic violence in contemporary China: Continuity and advances. *International Journal of Offender Therapy and Comparative Criminology*, *62*(16), 4879–4887.

Zhou, M. (2004). Assimilation, the Asian way. In T. Jacoby (Ed.), *Reinventing the melting pot: The new immigrants and what it means to be an American* (pp. 139–154). New York: Basic Books.

3 Cultural Beliefs, Mental Health, and Stigma

A Network Perspective

Social Networks in East Asian Cultures

Chapter 2 theoretically laid out the architecture of East Asian cultures and identified their most salient values and beliefs that impose upon experiences of mental health – for better or worse. In this chapter, I extend this theorization to examine how they manifest in the social networks that animate social life in East Asia. I discuss the ways that such networks facilitate the spread of stigma and mental health issues.

This network perspective fundamentally has several elements. People are connected to one another, which add up to building a network. Culture plays a significant role in determining the structure of social networks. In highly individualistic cultures like America, for instance, people are much more likely to be spread out. There, the culture valorizes individual achievement over collective achievements. Your successes are your own. People do not have the same sense of obligation to one another. These cultural principles filter down into the way people choose, build, and maintain their connections, which, in turn, come to be reflected in the structure of their networks. We may theorize a typical social network to look very much like Figure 3.1. Figure 3.1 shows a sample network graph or map of a network, where dots (or nodes) represent people and the lines between them (or edges) represent connections between people who know each other.

In East Asian cultures, by contrast, collectivism is the reigning imperative for interactions. As we observed in Chapter 2, people feel a greater sense of obligation and reciprocity to a larger social unit. Indeed, the status of an individual is linked to the status of their larger social unit. The family is perhaps the most significant of these social units, where the successes and failures of an individual are taken to reflect on the honor of the family itself. This pushes children to study hard and prize academic merits above their own health, women to perform traditional household duties and submissive gender roles, and men and women alike to suppress their emotions as a sign of maturity. In East Asian cultures that prize status and etiquette, this sense of obligation also extends beyond the

DOI:10.4324/9781003308720-3

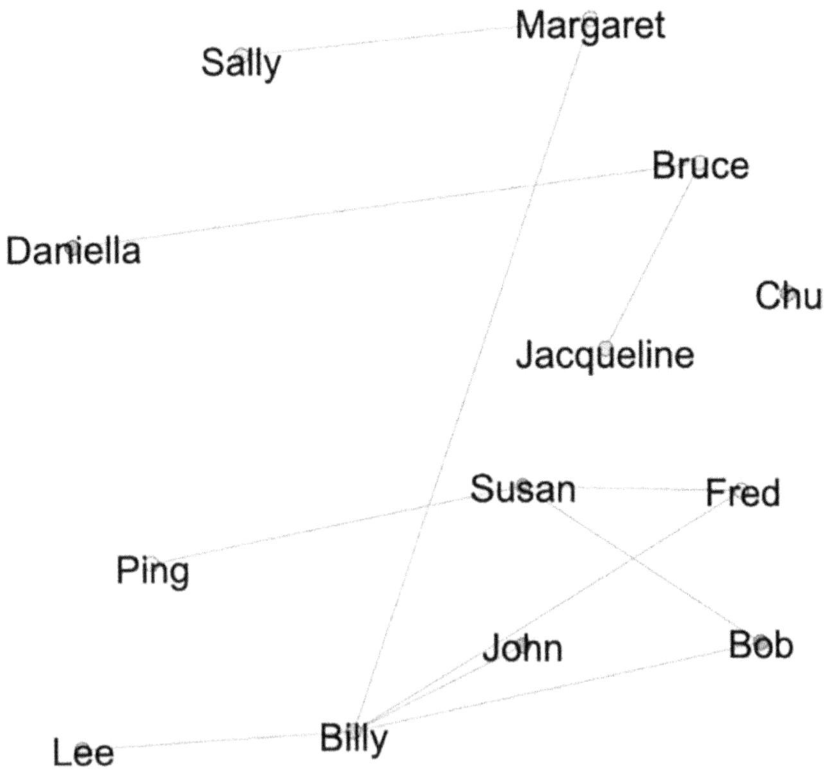

Figure 3.1 Exemplar Western social network.

family to friendship circles, peer groups, circles of work colleagues, and so on. How well someone abides by social etiquette powerfully reflects on their personal reputation (or *mianzi*). This brand of personal reputation is unique to East Asian cultures because they are entirely social, not institutional. Reputation is what orients actors within their connections and interactions with them – a mental ledger of the value of each person in a network, knowing whom to give to and receive from (Au, 2021).

The uniqueness of East Asian cultures sensitizes us to important structural qualities of social networks that have repercussions for the content of interactions within them. East Asian networks are *denser* and *grouped*, which make them look more like Figure 3.2.

Networks are denser in that out of the total number of possible connections within a network (where everyone knows everyone else), many of these connections are in fact real. As a matter of etiquette, people in East Asian cultures are often connected to a greater number of others in a social setting like school or the workplace. This surfaces in a

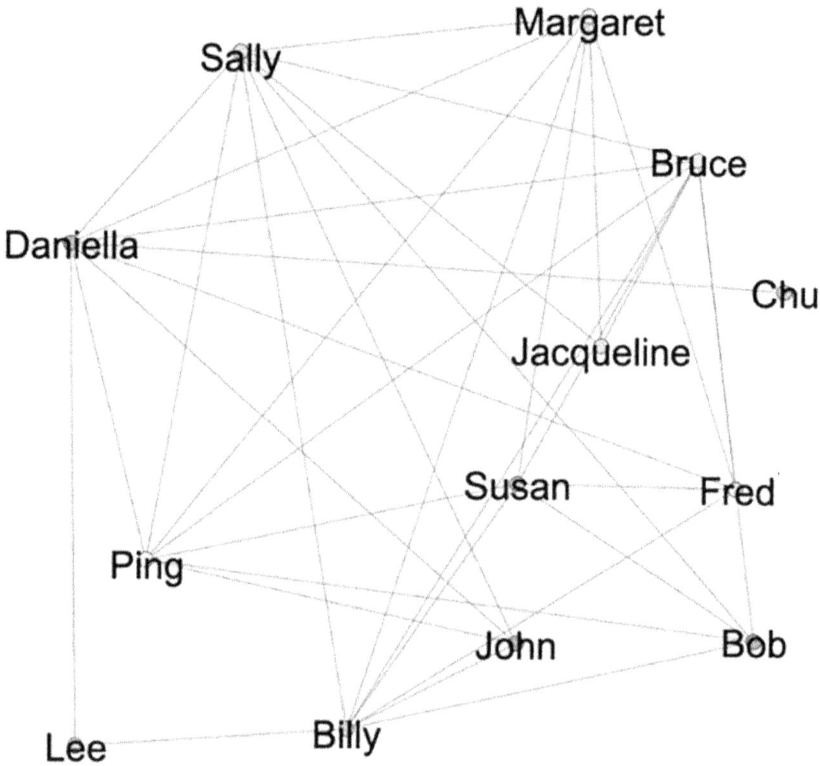

Figure 3.2 Exemplar East Asian social network.

greater number of interconnections within social networks, which, in turn, means that information flows faster within them. Since everyone is connected with a greater number of others, information travels faster and to greater expanses of the network.

The density and prevalence of groups in networks are also how the sense of obligation to a larger social unit is reinforced. Those who break faith from proper etiquette are very quickly found out by others and branded a person of poor quality – a disapproval that spreads through their networks to depreciate their reputation or *mianzi* (Hwang, 1987, pp. 960–961). Thus, East Asian cultural principles and their social network structure are mutually sustaining: people are driven to connect with others for the sake of etiquette, obligation, and their personal reputation, even if they are not very close with them. Once they are connected, they are then held to standards of etiquette, obligation, and personal reputation by the many eyes that watch them, because of how well connected they become.

In what follows, I discuss how this dialectic leads networks to influence mental health, as the structure of East Asian networks that sustains this sense of obligation to others and relational kind of personal status is also what ends up policing people for their mental health issues and spreads stigma.

Social Credentials and Resources Access in East Asian Networks

Social network scholarship asserts that social influence happens when people solicit normative guidance from and compare their own attitudes to those of a reference group who are close to us in some way (Erickson, 1988; Marsden & Friedkin, 1993). People perform better in work and life when they are better connected and are with better people, which is determined not only by the structural characteristics of the network (e.g., how dense its connections are or how transitive it is to allow information flow through it) but by personal characteristics about the agent. It is here that broader forms of inequality can emerge, such as when disadvantages are created by a person's location in a network or when advantages are created that preclude similar advantages from others.

Personal characteristics exert influence over a person's ability to network and benefit from their network through the interpersonal evaluation of what Nan Lin (2001a, p. 20) calls social credentials, which are an important resource that social capital provides – an endorsement of one's certifications by the relationships and ties that one has (Lin, 2001b). Social credentials mediate social influence by virtue of how networks operate as prisms. Podolny (2001) influentially asserts that networks diffract differences that reverberate through networks by providing information cues to observers based on the presence or absence of ties.

To illustrate, firms pick up on the presence (or absence) of a tie between two market actors as an informational cue to determine the quality of a potential partner and to decide whether or not to partner or invest in them (Podolny, 2001, p. 34). Similarly, social actors look to the (social, symbolic, economic, cultural, etc.) resources that someone possesses as well as whom they are connected with as cues to make inferences about the quality of an someone's social position (Lin, 2001a, p. 20, 2001b).

Thus, social credentials amplify not only the value of the information and referrals that one gives or receives but also the likelihood that one will receive them. People tend to assess another person's reputation and status before exchanging information, offering job information, giving referrals, or providing any sort of help. We do this to weather the uncertainty of how they might respond, determine the risk to personal reputation that comes from helping them, and decide whether they are worthy of help.

The evaluation of social credentials thus sustains inequality when it entangles prestige with personal characteristics, excluding those who do not possess whatever characteristics are valued in a network.

In East Asian cultures that have strong patriarchal values, respect for status, and stigmatization of mental health, covered in Chapter 2, this means that women and those with mental health issues (and especially women *with* mental health issues) are most at risk.

Gender is a prominent social characteristic where this inequality is most visible. A long tradition of social network scholarship has identified how women are associated with domestic housework, subordinate roles, and worse performances in the workplace. This means that the very same qualities that help men succeed, exert greater social influence, and gain access to novel information do not hold for women.

For example, the diversity of a person's networks is a quality that should improve the social resources an actor will receive. Consider person A who only has friends who are lawyers and person B who has friends who are lawyers, doctors, construction workers, painters, artists, and janitors. Person A will only ever have access to information provided by lawyers, all of whom will also very likely share the same kinds of information anyway, since their work and lifestyles are so similar. By contrast, person B will benefit from having sources of information in diverse sectors (Granovetter, 1973), will be more likely to know someone with the most appropriate resources to provide help when they need it (Lin et al., 2001), and will have greater visibility – a bird's eye view – of their networks in a way that allows them to exert influence over (or broker) how others in their network collaborate and share information (Burt, 2004).

Yet, Ron Burt (2005, 1992/2009) finds that even when a woman has diverse contacts within an organization, she must rely on a man's networks and leverage his contacts through him as a proxy to participate in collaborations. Much work since has identified how these correlations have remained true for women (network diversity being useful predominantly through men) and continue to present challenges to upward mobility, particularly among ethnic minorities (Brady, 2018; DiMaggio & Garip, 2012; Erickson, 2004; Rubineau & Fernandez, 2015). Kmec and colleagues (2010) discovered that when people take the initiative to help someone else find new jobs, the men are mostly moved into male-dominated, higher-paying work groups, whereas the women into female-dominated, lower-paying work groups in sustaining the typical segregation of a job market by gender.

Here, regardless of whether women are moved into male-dominated or female-dominated jobs, they obtain significantly worse-paying jobs and/or lower job rewards, such as job authority, than their male counterparts (Kmec et al., 2010). Erickson (2006) advances the argument by demonstrating how influence itself is weaker when it concerns women, such that men are less attentive to information concerning gender inequality, not taking it seriously until validated by multiple sources.

Just like how one's social credentials are weighted differently depending on their gender, so too are they assessed differently based on mental health problems. As a stigmatized condition, mental health problems may be seen to lower the status of an individual and their families in East Asian cultures.

This matters because individuals with mental health problems suffer a double whammy when it comes to their networks. In social networks, those with lower status are perceived to be less trustworthy by others – enough to restrict access to help when requested (Marin, 2012; Granovetter, 1995). Put differently, when individuals with mental health problems most need help, they are least likely to ask for it and the people around them are also least likely to help.

People are thus policed for their mental health by their networks. According to the latest China Mental Health Survey, less than 8% of individuals with major depressive disorder had ever sought any type of professional help in China – significantly lower than Western countries (Phillips et al., 2009; Kohn et al., 2004). This has owed to the stigmatization of mental health – and treatment – in East Asian cultures, rooted in discriminatory beliefs about mental health issues as a symptom of moral depravity and poverty (Lasalvia et al., 2013).

Those with higher statuses and reputation typically gain access to a greater wealth of social resources, like knowledge about informal rules of the office or information about a new kind of vitamin, that informally help them move up and experience better quality of life. People with higher reputations are evaluated to be of good moral standing that makes them a good person of choice for others to network with.

Furthermore, those with lower statuses also lose reputation and cultural resources that informally help upward mobility. Their value and reputation as a person of good moral standing makes them a poor person of choice for others to network with, cutting them off from their connections and the information they have (Erickson, 1996a, 2004). Those with lower statuses, like women and/or people with mental health issues, are more likely to be precluded from flows of help and information crucial for upward mobility (Marin, 2012; Smith, 2005). Taken together, this ultimately reinforces inequality when only those of a higher social class possess the social resources (i.e., information) through better education needed for upward mobility, disproportionately accumulating influence and information diffusion at the top.

Contagion in East Asian Networks

A social network perspective shows that illnesses can spread as quickly as they are felt (Hoge et al., 2017). Experiences of mental health are *contagious* in patterned ways. And these patterns tell a compelling story of a mental health epidemic on the rise in East Asia.

There are two kinds of contagion in social networks.

The first is *simple contagion*, which is the spread of information. Simple contagion may be thought of as how information about mental health illnesses about members spread. In East Asian cultures, cooperative norms encourage this type of contagion. Exchange happens more fluidly and frequently in bounded groups, where cooperative norms work to mandate reciprocity and sanction discord. It sustains the homophily that is common to groups, which largely benefits members by ensuring everyone acts as a pool of social support that more stably provides for their needs (Coleman, 1988; Burt, 2005, p. 6; Enns et al., 2008; Uehara, 1990). Community members form ties and sustain them in response to pressure for mutuality in relations and to alleviate fears of offending others, such that ties embedded in triads in organizations or groups are more likely to endure than nonembedded ones (Burt, 2004; McFarland et al., 2014; Wellman & Wortley, 1990).

This insulated bubble of exchange within a group where social cohesion best flourishes is made possible by closure, which effectively hardens the boundaries of a group by discouraging the addition of new members and restricting the circulation of resources within the group (Coleman, 1988). Closed networks create the trust, community, and security needed to enforce norms of generalized exchange, where giving support is strongly associated with receiving it (Uehara, 1990). Within highly bounded groups in East Asia, this sense of obligation creates a conformity that accelerates rapid information diffusion or simple contagion. Examples might include family, friend circles, or even work groups. The boundaries for these groups are more rigid and harder to pass through because of organizational constraints, such as working in the same workplace, and social ones, like membership in the same family. What results nonetheless is a higher bandwidth – speed and frequency – of contagion.

In exploring the novelty of the social network and e-mail content exchanged within an executive recruiting firm, Aral and Van Alstyne (2011) importantly reveal that strong ties have a higher rate of information flow and likelihood of novel information contained within this flow. What's more is they find that people *like* this higher information flow because there is deeper knowledge that they have about their connections. This, in turn, facilitates social exchanges of information that enable fellow group members to better help one another by finding out what needs they have and gaining access to greater diversity and novelty of information about different networks (Burt, 2005; Coleman, 1988; Erickson, 1996b, 2006; Small, 2009). So, people in East Asian cultures are incentivized to keep bandwidth high.

Yet, this connectivity poses a threat to people who experience mental health issues. Rumors, for instance, are found to spread so much faster on East Asian networks than other kinds of networks (Lai & Wong, 2002). The most striking feature of such simple contagion in East Asian networks is how quickly it spreads regardless of how strong or weak ties are and position in the network. Put differently, information not only spreads quickly within a given group but even has a greater likelihood of spreading quickly *across* groups. In fact, people who are farther removed from a person of interest in a network may even absorb and facilitate further spreads of information quicker, because they do not know the person and have less to lose with spreading a rumor (Min & San Miguel, 2018). Echoing this argument, a recent thrust in the network analysis of cultural production has been to demonstrate how peripheral members of a network glean from the structural advantage of having more weak ties in diverse network locations, fewer ties to the core, and more intransitivity, which is conducive to communication of new ideas (Cattani & Ferriani, 2008; De Vaan et al., 2015).

The second form of contagion is *complex contagion*, which is the spread of collective behaviors. Complex contagion diffuses things differently than simple contagion because it requires confirmation from different sources and relies on tie width, having more sources confirm the same information, more than tie length, or how close or far two people are in a network (Centola & Macy, 2007).

There are two things that complex contagion spreads in exacerbating mental health issues: (1) exclusion and inequality of victims, as well as (2) mental health problems themselves.

(1) The density of East Asian networks exacerbates complex contagion of excluding people with mental health issues. Since everyone is highly connected to many others in a given network, they are beholden to conform to complex contagion. Put differently, everyone is exposed to a large number of connections behaving in patterned ways, which largens the pressure to conform, rather than innovate or do anything differently. Just as actors are more likely to feel dissimilar and uncomfortable when they fail to adopt attitudes that others have (Van den Bulte & Lilien, 2001), they are more likely to *not* adopt new attitudes or include someone into a network when others have not.

The argument gains credence from Godart and Mears' (2009) work, evincing how the same group of fashion models monopolize all bookings and continue to do so because of creative directors located in the network core. At the core are actors who have the most prestige and so have the most to lose in terms of credentials. These actors remain wary of straying from an institutional framework of sedimented network-specific meanings and behaviors seen to be most common in the core (Comunian & England, 2019). This resonates with White's (2008, 2018) classic assessment of how firms replicate the status quo. Producers with higher prestige do not produce more innovative products because of the cohesive social influence processes at work in their common position in the core. Core producers' judgments often sway to normative pressures and so homogenize, ultimately moving production away from innovation and toward replication of the status quo of a market profile.

Thus, the behavior of ostracizing others with mental health issues to preserve one's own status spreads like wildfire. This is a fact that also prevents people with mental health problems from sharing their issues. In a study of how people with depression interact with their social networks, Schaefer and colleagues (2011) find that people who are depressed withdraw from their networks for fear of burdening their connections. Even more striking is that the people who do withdraw are actively marginalized by others in the network, who try to avoid them. In general, stigma is a barrier to the treatment and discussion of depression and other mental illnesses (Defreitas et al., 2018; Sun et al., 2019).

When depressed individuals then attempt to return to their networks, they are *blocked*, unwanted by others who do not wish to be associated with the stigma of mental health issues. The only people that depressed individuals can network with are reduced to others with depression, fellow outcasts marginalized by their networks. Thus, the conformity to larger group norms in East Asian cultures that diffuses information quickly in networks also diffuses the behavior of excluding others who have fallen in status, including people with mental health issues.

(2) Poor mental health, such as distress, depression, and anxiety, can spread subconsciously through social interactions like a virus. This complex contagion can be short-term. People reflect observations of others' moods and negative emotional states onto themselves. We see this most clearly in emergencies when someone's panic triggers a chain reaction in others, or even when we feel the urge to cry upon seeing others cry in-person or through recordings (Wild et al., 2001).

This complex contagion can also be long-term. When receiving and processing others' negative interpretations of events, individuals can come to adopt them as well (Eisenberg et al., 2013). I never thought much about grading one assignment for a course I co-taught till a colleague droned on about how it was a *chore*. The following year, when I taught the same course, the thought crept up on me as I went to grade. Without knowing, a wisp of doubt flickered into existence – I had retained my colleague's sentiment and my motivation to grade wavered, even if for a moment and by a little.

Particular mental illnesses spread this way as well, such as depression and anxiety. This is common among spouses who share the same life challenges. A married person who gets laid off brings financial hardships for their entire household, and so the entire family grows more likely to experience depression. The structure of East Asian networks predisposes such illnesses to spread even faster. Comparing the contagion of mental health illnesses in youth in America versus Japan, for instance, we observe that contagion is minimal at best in America, but more in Japan.

Suicide ideation and depression are found to trigger a significant amount of attention on social media, to the effect of normalizing – and spreading – these illnesses (Carlyle et al., 2018). In particular, the etiquette of conformity and reciprocity in East Asian cultures fosters a digital culture that encourages copy-cat behaviors that facilitate complex contagion (Niederkrotenthaler et al., 2009).

Complex contagion has especially been prevalent amid the COVID-19 pandemic. East Asia witnessed the most stringent lockdown regimes in the world. As a result, people in the region were isolated for a longer period of time and forced to shift a greater proportion of their work and social life to online. Complex contagion spreads faster in the COVID-19 pandemic because everyone is exposed to a similar set of stressors. If we think of this in terms of the stress process model outlined in Chapter 1, the pandemic represents a macro-level stressor – something on the order of a nation that blankets the entire population. It might even be said to be a global stressor, since it has affected populations worldwide. Nonetheless, the wide-reaching influence of a pandemic is felt financially in the loss of income and employment, socially in the deprivation from the ability to socialize, emotionally within the family in terms of relationships, all of which comes to predispose people to depression, anxiety, and suicide ideation.

Witnessing someone else crumble to the pandemic has a deleterious effect on your own mental health, given that many of the same circumstances are shared in a pandemic. We might consider this in terms of the East Asian network in Figure 3.2. If Susan succumbs to the distress of losing her job, cooped up in a lockdown, and being unable to see her family, this is at once witnessed by Margaret, Bob, Ping, and Fred. These four are then just one conversation away from spreading this to Daniella, Sally, Bruce, John, and Billy. In just two steps, information about Susan's distress, and more importantly, the emotional gravity of the circumstances she represents, spreads through nearly the entire circuitry of her network. This is true for men as much as women in East Asian networks, both of whom are beholden to norms that suppress and stigmatize mental health, even when distressed.

Mental Health Segregation and Broader Inequality in East Asian Networks

The network exclusion of people with mental health issues on an interpersonal level has repercussions on how networks are structured at an aggregate or societal level. Such networking behaviors will tend to motivate people to make more exclusive networking choices and form clusters of homophilous subgroups based on preference (McFarland et al., 2014). People who prefer to network with others who do not have mental health issues will add up to create segregated clusters of people without mental health issues, separate from those with mental health illnesses.

These segregations can recursively spiral out to effect network closure at a macro level, giving rise to observations like that of DiPrete et al. (2011): the strongest predictors of connecting in the general population are social characteristics. Social support flows *within* these groups, but not across them. This creates many forms of inequality that disadvantage people with mental health issues, when groups without mental health issues are reputationally believed to possess higher status and attract more trust and resources, whereas those with mental health issues do not.

Morris (2004), for instance, finds that collectivistic villages that have more status are privy to having more connections that invite more information to prevent risk of disease (p. 214) and access to vaccines (p. 192). In the modern labor market, we observe similar kinds of inequality between the haves and have-nots.

In labor markets, networks act as pipes to exchange resources and prisms to differentiate others, through which information flows for firms and actors to make evaluations of each other based on the quality of goods and volume they produce, which produces an ordering of status that cues their identities (White, 2008; Podolny, 1993). In East Asia, the quality of firms depends less on the successes of the firm itself, and more on the personal status of the agents who represent their firms (Wu, 2018). Once more, we observe the prevalence of cultural beliefs that associate personal status with the status of one's larger social unit and personal ability to fulfill their obligations to such social units.

Closer analysis of labor markets shows how personal reputation comes to affect life chances for individuals and firms alike by affecting perceptions of uncertainty. Podolny (2001) shows that networks with more high-status firms tend to invest in established markets with more altercentric uncertainty – we know their performance records but not how others will react. In a similar vein, artistic producers in a competitive cultural market are not keen to collaborate with just anyone within the same sector of their work organization, but only with those they have already worked with in the past (Uzzi & Spiro, 2005). Thus, competition creates uncertainty in contexts such that information flows to those actors with advantages in network positions and in status, and, as a result, replicates inequality in a network by allowing a monopoly of information and cumulative advantages in market performance.

Within individual firms, status matters just as much, particularly since they are often structured hierarchically in ways that enable the higher status to oppress those lower. Work settings are rank-ordered according to status and class. Higher positions have greater access to and control of whatever the valued resources are "not only because more valued resources are intrinsically attached to that position, but also because of the position's greater accessibility to positions at other (primarily lower) rankings" (Lin, 2001a, p. 56). Ultimately, the workers who occupy positions up top hold a monopoly over the exchange of valued resources in the firm, sustained by advantages in control and resources that come from a higher position. Burt et al. (2018) identify strong trust in East Asian entrepreneurial networks, but they can just as easily lend for *domination* when managers leverage the weight of their position to manipulate flows of information and the direction of collaborations in structural holes (Burt, 2004). Moreover, senior managers can also bring to bear their superior knowledge of intrafirm business culture to maintain these advantages and monopolize their privileges using their position (Erickson, 1996a).

Thus, the suppression of emotionality and mental health issues is reinforced when a prototypical hierarchical company that mandates loyalty to the status quo and corporate policy by way of a performance network effect, wherein people adopt something for fear of losing out when they see prior adoptions by many or influential actors (Van den Bulte & Lilien, 2001). Mental health illnesses are forced into hiding and exacerbated by the structure of the modern labor market, where association with mental illness lowers one's status and ability to fit into the broader ecology of work.

Data from the 2017 Chinese General Social Survey by the National Natural Science Foundation of China (2017) (the latest iteration of a nationally representative dataset of the general population China) helps visualize this picture. Let us consider the proportion of the general population who, among those who *would* seek social support for emotional needs, report as their first-choice family and friends.

I find that just about three-quarters of people chose family, and about a fifth of people chose friends. This does not mean that people will seek help for mental health issues, neither does it mean that discussion of emotional issues translates to recognition of mental health issues. Rather, on average, it appears that most people in China who *would* seek emotional support would do so from family, then from friends. This signifies the hierarchy of status that lords over the workplace as a social space and the labor market in general, where emotions and mental health are banished concepts.

Though the discussion of mental health is burgeoning in corporate cultures in the West, this zeitgeist has yet to make its way to East Asia. This is reflected in stringent working conditions that have been the subject of media headlines in recent years. A prominent example is the "9–9–6" schedule in China, which refers to a start time at 9 AM, finishing time at 9 PM, and repeated over six days. Despite the distress and strain this practice causes to workers, it has nevertheless been a standard in many industries in the nation, including information and technology, finance, and other services sectors. A similar issue has been found in Japan, where white-collar workers, especially junior ones, are forced to work double-digit hours for extended periods of time. In addition, they are beholden to a hidden curriculum of success that mandates they spend their free time socializing with colleagues and superiors, often going out to bars with them after said double-digit-hour shifts. So pervasive and strenuous is this problem that many such workers have been found dead, collapsed in the streets with no preexisting condition and with such frequency that a term has been coined for this cause of death – *karoshi*.

No safe space exists for these workers, pushed to produce with little regard for their mental health. Thus, inequality in mental health (between those who have mental health issues issue and those who do not) replicates itself across multiple dimensions of work and social life in the labor market, as the demands of status and conformity pressure people – even those with mental health issues themselves – to suppress the subjects of mental health and emotionality.

Networks are the fabric of everyday life. But as this chapter shows, they work differently for different people based on the evaluation of their social credentials, interpretively linked to their personal characteristics. It is here that inequality arises, when individuals effect inequality by selectively choosing to associate with those in possession of a desired quality, setting up boundaries, and precluding those who do not; when, by free will or by obedience to cooperative norms, the privileged conform to preserve their advantages; or when people in more privileged status and network positions rely on domination to maintain their privileges.

References

Aral, S., & Van Alstyne, M. (2011). The diversity-bandwidth trade-off. *American Journal of Sociology*, *117*(1), 90–171.

Au, A. (2021). Guanxi 2.0: The exchange of likes in social networking sites. *Information, Communication & Society*, *24*(13), 1891–1906.

Brady, J. (2018). Toward a critical, feminist sociology of expertise. *Journal of Professions and Organization*, *5*(2), 123–138.

Burt, R. S. (2004). Structural holes and good ideas. *American Journal of Sociology*, *110*, 349–399.

Burt, R. S. (2005). *Brokerage and closure*. New York: Oxford University Press.

Burt, R. S. (2009). *Structural holes: The social structure of competition*. Cambridge, MA: Harvard University Press. (Original work published 1992)

Burt, R. S., Bian, Y., & Opper, S. (2018). More or less Guanxi: Trust is 60% network context, 10% individual difference. *Social Networks*, *54*, 12–25.

Carlyle, K., Guidry, J., Williams, K., Tabaac, A., & Perrin, P. (2018). Suicide conversations on Instagram™: Contagion or caring? *Journal of Communication in Healthcare*, *11*(1), 12–18.

Cattani, G., & Ferriani, S. (2008). A core/periphery perspective on individual creative performance: Social networks and cinematic achievements in the Hollywood film industry. *Organization Science*, *19*, 824–844.

Centola, D., & Macy, M. (2007). Complex contagion and the weakness of long ties. *American Journal of Sociology*, *113*, 702–734.

Coleman, J. (1988). Social capital in the creation of human capital. *American Journal of Sociology*, *94*, S95–S120.

Comunian, R., & England, L. (2019). Creative clusters and the evolution of knowledge and skills: From industrial to creative glassmaking. *Geoforum*, *99*, 238–224.

Defreitas, S., Crone, T., Deleon, M., & Ajayi, A. (2018). Perceived and personal mental health stigma in Latino and African American college students. *Front Public Health*, 6, Article 49.

De Vaan, M., Stark, D., & Vedres, B. (2015). Game changer: The topology of creativity. *American Journal of Sociology*, *120*, 1144–1194.

DiMaggio, P., & Garip, F. (2012). Network effects and social inequality. *Annual Review of Sociology*, *38*, 93–118.

DiPrete, T. A., Gelman, A., McCormick, T., Teitler, J., & Zheng, T. (2011). Segregation in social networks based on acquaintanceship and trust. *American Journal of Sociology, 116*(4), 1234–1283.

Eisenberg, D., Golberstein, E., Whitlock, J. L., & Downs, M. F. (2013). Social contagion of mental health: Evidence from college roommates. *Health Economics*, *22*(8), 965–986.

Enns, S., Malinick, T., & Matthews, R. (2008). It's not only who you know, it's also where they are: Using the position generator to investigate the structure of access to embedded resources. In N. Lin & B. H. Erickson (Eds.), *Social capital: An international research program* (pp. 255–281). Oxford: Oxford University Press.

Erickson, B. (1988). The relational basis of attitudes. In B. Wellman & S. Berkowitz (Eds.), *Social structures* (pp. 99–121). New York: Cambridge University Press.

Erickson, B. (1996a). The structure of ignorance. *Connections*, *19*(1), 28–38.

Erickson, B. (1996b). Culture, class, and connections. *American Journal of Sociology*, *102*, 217–251.

Erickson, B. (2004). The distribution of gendered social capital in Canada. In H. Flap & B. Volker (Eds.), *Creation and returns of social capital: A new research program* (pp. 27–50). New York: Routledge.

Erickson, B. (2006). Persuasion and perception: New models of network effects on gendered issues. In B. O'Neill & E. Gidengil (Eds.), *Gender and social capital* (pp. 293–322). New York: Routledge.

Godart, F., & Mears, A. (2009). How do cultural producers make creative decisions? Lessons from the catwalk. *Social Forces*, *88*, 671–692.

Granovetter, M. S. (1973). The strength of weak ties. *American Journal of Sociology*, *78*(6), 1360–1380.

Granovetter, M. S. (1995). *Getting a job: A study of contacts and careers* (2nd ed.). Chicago, IL: University of Chicago Press.

Hoge, C. W., Ivany, C. G., & Adler, A. B. (2017). Suicidal behaviors within army units: Contagion and implications for public health interventions. *JAMA Psychiatry*, *74*(9), 871–872.

Hwang, K. (1987). Face and favor: The Chinese power game. *American Journal of Sociology*, *92*(4), 944–974.

Kmec, J. A., McDonald, S., & Trimble, L. B. (2010). Making gender fit and "correcting" gender misfits: Sex segregated employment and the non-search process. *Gender & Society*, *24*(2), 213–236.

Kohn, R., Saxena, S., Levav, I., & Saraceno, B. (2004). The treatment gap in mental health care. *Bulletin of the World Health Organization*, *82*, 858–866.

Lai, G., & Wong, O. (2002). The tie effect on information dissemination: The spread of a commercial rumor in Hong Kong. *Social Networks*, *24*, 49–75.

Lasalvia, A., Zoppei, S., Van Bortel, T., Bonetto, C., Cristofalo, D., Wahlbeck, K., Bacle, S., Van Audenhove, C., van Weeghel, J., Reneses, B., Germanavicius, A., Economou, M., Lanfredi, M., Sartorius, N., Lopez-Ibor, J., Thornicroft, G., & The ASPEN/INDIGO Study Group. (2013). Global pattern of experienced and anticipated discrimination reported by people with major depressive disorder: A cross-sectional survey. *Lancet*, *381*, 55–62.

Lin, N. (2001a). *Social capital: A theory of social structure and action*. Cambridge, MA: Cambridge University Press.

Lin, N. (2001b). Building a network theory of social capital. In N. Lin, K. Cook, & R. Burt (Eds.), *Social capital: Theory and research* (pp. 3–30). New York: Aldine de Gruyter.

Lin, N., Fu, Y., & Hsung, R. (2001). The position generator: Measurement techniques for investigations of social capital. In N. Lin, K. Cook, & R. Burt (Eds.), *Social capital: Theory and research* (pp. 57–81). New York: Aldine de Gruyter.

Marin, A. (2012). Don't mention it: Why people don't share job information, when they do, and why it matters. *Social Networks*, *34*(2), 181–192.

Marsden, P. V., & Friedkin, N. E. (1993). Network studies of social influence. *Sociological Methods & Research*, *22*(1), 127–151.

McFarland, D. A., Moody, J., Diehl, D., Smith, J. A., & Thomas, R. J. (2014). Network ecology and adolescent social structure. *American Sociological Review*, *79*(6), 1088–1121.

Min, B., & San Miguel, M. (2018). Competing contagion processes: Complex contagion triggered by simple contagion. *Scientific Reports*, *8*(1), 1–8.

Morris, M. (2004). *Network epidemiology: A handbook for survey design and data collection*. Oxford: Oxford University Press.

National Natural Science Foundation of China. 中国综合社会调查. (2017). *Chinese general social survey 2017*. Beijing: National Natural Science Foundation of China. Retrieved from www.cnsda.org/index.php?r=projects/view&id=94525591

Niederkrotenthaler, T., Till, B., Kapusta, N., Voracek, M., Dervic, K., & Sonneck, G. (2009). Copycat effects after media reports on suicide: A population-based ecologic study. *Social Science & Medicine*, *69*(7), 1085–1090.

Phillips, M., Zhang, J., Shi, Q., Song, Z., Ding, Z., Pang, S., Li, X., Zhang, Y., & Wang, Z. (2009). Prevalence, treatment, and associated disability of mental disorders in four provinces in China during 2001–05: An epidemiological survey. *Lancet*, *373*, 2041–2053.

Podolny, J. M. (1993). A status-based model of market competition. *American Journal of Sociology*, *98*(4), 829–872.

Podolny, J. M. (2001). Networks as the pipes and prisms of the market. *American Journal of Sociology*, *107*, 33–60.

Rubineau, B., & Fernandez, R. M. (2015). Tipping points: The gender segregating and desegregating effects of network recruitment. *Organization Science*, *26*(6), 1646–1664.

Schaefer, D. R., Kornienko, O., & Fox, A. M. (2011). Misery does not love company: Network selection mechanisms and depression homophily. *American Sociological Review*, *76*(5), 764–785.

Small, M. (2009). *Unanticipated gains: Origins of network inequality in everyday life*. Chicago, IL: University of Chicago Press.

Smith, S. S. (2005). "Don't put my name on it": Social capital activation and job-finding assistance among the black urban poor. *American Journal of Sociology*, *111*(1), 1–57.

Sun, Y., Chen, G., Wang, L., Li, N., Srisurapanont, M., Hong, J. P., Hatim, A., Chen, C., Udomratn, P., Nam Bae, J., Fang, Y., Chua, C., Liu, S., George, T., Bautista, D., Chan, E., Rosh, J., Yang, H., Su, Y., & Si, T. (2019). Perception of stigma and its associated factors among patients with major depressive disorder: A multicenter survey from an Asian population. *Frontiers in Psychiatry*, *10*, Article 321.

Uehara, E. (1990). Dual exchange theory, social networks, and informal social support. *American Journal of Sociology*, *96*(3), 521–557.

Uzzi, B., & Spiro, J. (2005). Collaboration and creativity: The small world problem. *American Journal of Sociology*, *111*(2), 447–504.

Van den Bulte, C., & Lilien, G. L. (2001). Medical innovation revisited: Social contagion versus marketing effort. *American Journal of Sociology*, *106*(5), 1409–1435.

Wellman, B., & Wortley, S. (1990). Different strokes from different folks: Community ties and social support. *American Journal of Sociology*, *96*(3), 558–588.

White, H. C. (2008). *Identity and control: How social formations emerge*. Princeton, NJ: Princeton University Press.

White, H. C. (2018). *Markets from networks*. Princeton, NJ: Princeton University Press.

Wild, B., Erb, M., & Bartels, M. (2001). Are emotions contagious? Evoked emotions while viewing emotionally expressive faces: Quality, quantity, time course and gender differences. *Psychiatry Research*, *102*(2), 109–124.

Wu, B. (2018). From individual social capital to collective social capital: Empirical evidence from inter-firm financing trust network. *Journal of Chinese Sociology*, *5*(1), Article 18.

4 Cultural Beliefs and Social Support

The Boons of Social Support

"Ask and you shall be given" goes the verse 7:7 in the book of Matthew in the Bible (English Standard Version Bible, 2001, Matthew 7:7). Behind one of the most widely cited phrases is an important sociological concept and a classic cornerstone of scholarship in network science and sociology: social support. The idea behind the Psalm holds true in most areas of social life. At no point does one venture through the life course in work, family life, social life, without the need to call on another for some kind of help. Those who do not have help at those critical junctures are less likely to make it through the hurdle.

Of the types of coping resources for mental health issues available, social support is arguably one of the most important. Social support spans various types, as will be discussed, but is fundamentally the "perception or experience that one is loved and cared for by others, esteemed and valued, and part of a social network of mutual assistance and obligations" (Wills, 1991 cited by Taylor, 2011, p. 192). This definition captures the fact that social support need not only be the explicit provision of help but the perception of its availability in the first place (Dour et al., 2014; Thoits, 1995). The tremendous benefits of social support for mental health have been consistently documented by a large body of scholarship.

Researchers have found that social support reduces psychological distress related to depression, anxiety, chronically stressful conditions, such as terminal illnesses, and traumatic events. Social support goes further to even protect against cognitive decline, heart disease, and other physical health ailments. In fact, longitudinal research studies on social support have found that it is one of the most power predictors of longevity and good health, perhaps even more so than traditional lifestyle choices and risks like exercise, obesity, diet, and lipids (House et al., 1988; MacDonald, 2007). People who have higher quality and quantity of relationships are also at lower risk of early death, debilitating feelings of isolation, and poor mental health in general (Alsubaie et al., 2019; Chrostek et al., 2016; Herbst-Damm & Kulik, 2005; VanKim & Nelson, 2013; Wang et al., 2018).

DOI:10.4324/9781003308720-4

Social support helps us in an instrumental sense when we receive the help we need to overcome a challenge we encounter, but the fundamental blueprint of how it helps our mental health is fascinating. Philosophically, it works by speaking to a fundamental human condition of sociality, where all the structures that permeate our lives since time immemorial have been relational in nature – built through and for communion with others. Psychologically, it operates by satisfying what appear to be inherent desires for sociality, attention, and visibility. Social support for older adults, for instance, helps prevent loneliness and cognitive decline by offering a source of psychological stimulation and encouragement for participation in voluntary and physical activities (Kuiper et al., 2016; Piolatto et al., 2022).

We glimpse the significance of sociality empirically in the fact that providing social support for someone else may create beneficial health effects for the help-giver as much as the receiver (Brown et al., 2003; Taylor, 2011). Explanations for why this happens fall into the terrain of altruistic behaviors, where people want to help because they like helping (Schnall et al., 2010). East Asian cultures emphasize the family as the primordial group to which one belongs, which tends to enhance this tendency of altruism. People want to help their kin because they are their kin.

It may even be argued that the provision of and need for social support are programmed into us. A large-scale study of nationally representative longitudinal samples in the U.S. population found that social support has biochemical roots. The study traced key biomarkers that regulate our physiological health and found that people who participated more frequently in social activities and received social support from others had lower risks across the board (Yang et al., 2013; Yang et al., 2016). Conversely, people who were less active on these fronts had a higher risk of inflammation, cardiovascular disease, and even cancer (Penwell & Larkin, 2010).

Social support has been usefully broken down by scholars into different taxonomies of type, channels of provision, circumstances, how identity matters in its exchange, and network consequences. Focusing on the cultural emphasis on family described in Chapter 2 as well as network and social structure of embeddedness outlined in Chapter 3, a cultural perspective enlightens us to how these differences distinguish East Asian cultures.

Embeddedness and Tiered Trust

There are two kinds of social support that Nan Lin (2001a, p. 20, 2001b) classically outlined in his eponymous book *Social Capital*: instrumental support and expressive support. Instrumental support refers to the provision of resources to do with positions and statuses, embedded within a hierarchical organizational structure such as in a labor market. Job information, referrals, and other kinds of job help are some of the most common examples of instrumental support. Expressive support, by contrast, consists of the provision of emotional help and satisfaction of emotional needs. A friend who makes time to spend time with and console someone going through a bad break-up is one such form of expressive support.

Who is most likely to give help when asked? For Western cultures like in the United States and Canada, the answer is variable. Plickert et al. (2007) find in a network study of Canadians residing close to Toronto that kinship ties are not, in fact, more likely than friends to be reciprocally supportive. In particular, they find that friends might provide less variety of support than do kin, but they surprisingly provided more than kin, especially extended kin (Wellman & Wortley, 1990).

Friends, furthermore, were most apt at providing expressive or emotional support when called upon (Miller & Darlington, 2002). Identity also mattered in terms of gender, where women reported expressing themselves emotionally more often and they provided more emotional support. This is consistent with other network and sociological studies that take stock of gendered socialization, such that women are socialized into society differently than their male counterparts (Brody & Hall, 2010; Wellman & Frank, 2001). That is, women are led to adopt different expectations about their roles as supportive actors in the household, family, and workplace and, as a result, are looked upon as intimate caretakers.

Western cultures are predicated on the exchange of both expressive and instrumental support. It is common for both forms of support to be exchanged in personal networks, with little regard for distinctions between, say, kinship and non-kinship ties. East Asian cultures, by contrast, have myriad contingencies that complicate the exchange of social support, a lot of which involves the identity of the people on both the giving and receiving ends.

Recalling from Chapter 2, however, East Asian cultures differ in the deep obligations that one has to a larger social unit. This primordially begins with the family, before fanning out to include other social units. This ordering is formally visualized in Figure 4.1.

Figure 4.1 is an exemplar prototype for the ordering of networks in a person's life in East Asian cultures based on their relationship with them. China's first sociologist Fei Xiaotong (1947/1992) also wrote very influentially about this ordering, noting that network structures of personal networks in China manifest in the appearance of concentric circles that ripple out like a stone dropped into a body of water. This is a useful heuristic for understanding Figure 4.1 as an illustration of a person's networks. A given person is assumed to be in the center of the circles. Rippling out are rings or categories that indicate tie strength (how close a tie is to someone) under which their ties fall under. The rings closest to

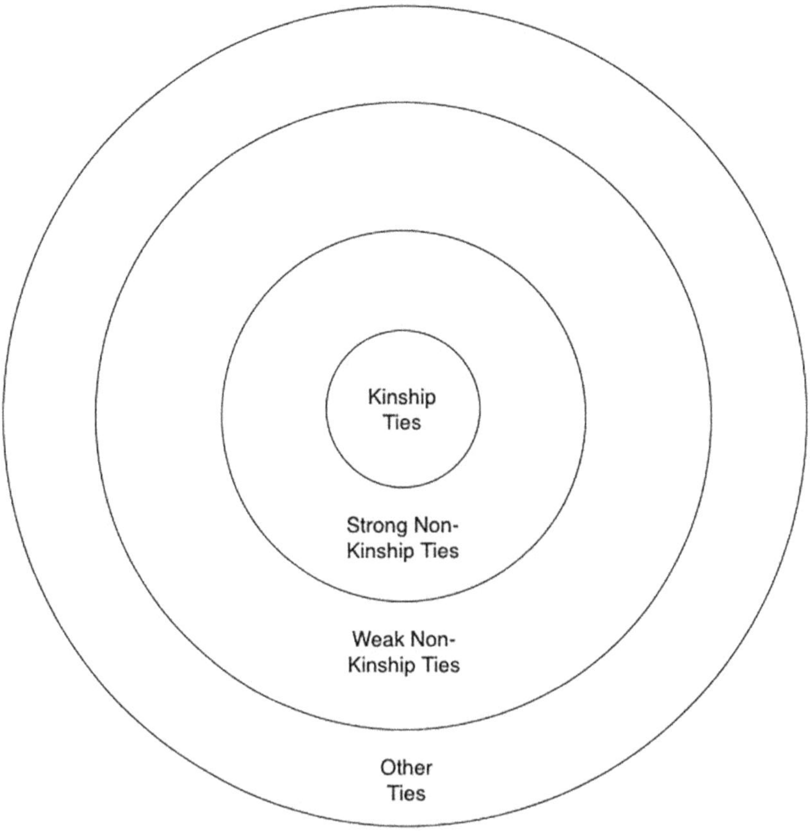

Figure 4.1 A model of ties and trust in a person's network, tiered in concentric circles.

the center are the strongest. The greater the distance from the center, the weaker the tie.

Naturally, then, the rings are not merely nominal but have real-world consequences for social support. As Chapter 2 described, East Asian cultures are defined by a sense of obligation. The ordering we see in Figure 4.1 is thus also a road map or guide for who a person can ask for help from and for what. Unlike in Western cultures, kinship ties are the default, go-to source of support. One is expected to be tightknit with their family.

Kinship ties in East Asia more broadly may even serve as a primary source of welfare, reflecting what Nauck and Arránz Becker (2013) observe in a cross-national study to be a general pattern of tightknit relationships among kinship ties – that is comparatively rare in Western nations. They go further to pinpoint the roots of this tightknit kinship pattern in the extended household living arrangements common to such cultures.

If one does not seek help from family, it may even reflect poorly on their own reputation as unfilial. Conversely, one is also expected to help their family, with the same risk to their reputation if they do not. In China, for instance, people may expect more support from their children than even from their spouses (Cong & Silverstein, 2011).

Thus, where friendship might work better for social support in Western cultures because friends are normatively bound on a voluntary basis, family is the social support of choice in East Asian cultures. The reason is different, yet the same. People more actively maintain friendship ties in Western cultures and kinship ties in East Asian cultures because their respective cultural norms compel them to conceive of reputation in this manner (Wellman & Wortley, 1990; Crohan & Antonucci, 1989).

It follows, therefore, that trust is tiered and highly centralized in East Asian cultures. This echoes the embeddedness described in Chapter 3, where people who are part of the same networks are more likely to know and exchange more often with each other. Here, we realize that this embeddedness is intensified in certain rings of a network, namely, with kinship ties. We see further evidence of this in how people use ties of different strengths in East Asian cultures. A consensus holds in Western network scholarship that weak ties are more useful for a variety of purposes. This is because weak ties are hypothesized to permit access to more diverse sources of information, as Chapter 3 alluded. This diversity also invigorates the reliance on social friendships as sources of social companionship (Plickert et al., 2007; Uehara, 1990, 1995; Wellman & Frank, 2001).

East Asian networks are not so entrepreneurial. Cultural expectations about the significance of communities push individuals toward strong ties instead. Yanjie Bian (1997) observed as much in his classic work on the Chinese labor market, finding that strong ties are the most helpful in securing help from job-assigning authorities as well as acting as intermediaries to connect job-seekers with higher-paying jobs of better fit than those who did not rely on strong ties.

In terms of mental health, this embeddedness lends well to fostering novel *channels* of social support in East Asian cultures. We observe what network scientists call generalized exchange and restricted exchange. Generalized exchange refers to exchange within a social unit, where fellow members help one another through and simply because they are part of the same social unit, less so because of their specific identities. Person A may provide help to person B, and receive help in return from person C, all of whom belong to the same group. Restricted exchange refers to dyadic exchanges, or one-on-one exchanges between two individuals on the basis of their identities. Person A gives and receives help from person B in more of a tit-for-tat fashion.

Information is a common social resource with which these channels are used to fire off help. In East Asian cultures, group members are quick to disseminate information to other members in communal settings, sharing it with entire groups at the same time. Social media notably catalyzes this effect as people gain the structural ability to join chatrooms and group discussions where every member has real-time access to conversations had within the group, as Chapter 3 discussed.

Though East Asian cultures may repress emotionality, as discussed in Chapter 2, the rich channels of generalized and restricted exchange alternatively mean that existing networks are very apt at offering instrumental support. The combination of densely embedded networks, especially with kinship ties, and instrumental support may be an antidote to work-related challenges. Yanjie Bian's (1997) labor market study in China is a good example.

Examinations of the Japanese and Korean General Social Surveys, statistically representative datasets on the general populations of Japan and Korea respectively, corroborate the same idea. Japanese and Korean people are found to rank their non-kin ties hierarchically, as either "superior" or "inferior" to themselves. Thinking of one's ties in instrumentalist terms appears to carry instrumental benefits of a similar kind. People who have more "superior" ties, for instance, benefit from being more politically active (Bian & Ikeda, 2018).

In my own examination of the latest 2012 Japanese General Social Survey, I find that instrumental social support remains very important in overcoming instrumental challenges, such as finding a job. When asked to name how many people helped in the process of getting their current or last job, such as by putting in a good word or passing along information, the average number of people who job-seekers relied upon for help was just over two. When asked to answer whether this kind of help is important for finding a job, over 90% responded yes out of everyone who responded.

Let us consider also the case of the largest labor market in East Asia, China, using the Chinese General Social Survey, which is a statistically representative survey of the Chinese general population. About 15.85% of the Chinese general population reported relying on strong ties (family and close friends) for work-related issues, and 11% reported relying on weak ties (everyone else) for work-related issues. People rely tremendously on their ties for resolving issues.

However, I urge caution about overestimating the protective effects of work help for mental health. It is one thing to have help when it comes to overcoming work-related challenges, but it is entirely another thing to say that this help also protects individual mental health from the stress of facing work-related challenges in the first place.

My analysis of the Chinese General Social Survey indicates much the same concern about the limits of such help for mental health. I built statistical models using help from weak ties and help from strong ties for work-related issues as independent variables and regressed them against life happiness as a dependent variable. I controlled for the effects of demographic variables such as education, income, gender, and age. Ultimately, I found that the main effects of help from weak *and* strong ties alike were both insignificant on how happy respondents felt.

This brushes upon the idea of satisfaction with social support. It is higher satisfaction with social support that significantly reduces depressive symptoms and other symptoms of mental health illnesses (Schacter & Margolin, 2019); merely having social support may not be enough to do the trick. While we may infer that there is not so much satisfaction in my aggregate-level analysis, it is worth noting that there is direct measure of mental health symptoms in the Chinese General Social Survey and that there is alternative evidence of satisfaction with social support in smaller-scale studies in the nation (Tengku Mohd et al., 2019; Tsai et al., 2005).

In this manner, patterns of tightknit kinship ties in East Asian cultures also bring with them unique forms of social support that would be sanctioned in Western cultures. American poet Ocean Vuong (2019) said evocatively of the subtlety that defines Asian communication:

> What I learned from these [Asian] refugee women is you don't have to talk it out. That's the great Western myth, you know. "You gotta talk it out," "you gotta get it there," "lay it all out," and I think when I see them, they're more invested in the present. The wounds are understood and sometimes even language can't hash them all out. They taught me that despite what happened, I can still be of use to you. So, when I see you, it's "are you hungry?" "What can I do?" There's a wisdom in accepting what happened is beyond your control. They never asked for their country to be bombed. They never asked for their husbands who abused them. But what they can do is say, "regardless of what happened, I care for you, and I'm gonna find a way to keep caring for you." That's what I learned.

Vuong's lyrical recollection of the women in his life limns the subtlety of expression and care in (East) Asian cultures. Rather than tackling issues head-on as we might expect in Western cultures, people are depicted in Vuong's account to speak around trauma, to nurse scars more than address their causes. Implicit in Vuong's account is also the idea that people do not share about deeply personal issues to save face, as Chapter 2 discussed.

Nonetheless, there are myriad benefits to such cultural norms of subtlety in expression that are scientific as much as they are poetic. In network science, they reflect a type of social support called nonsearching. Nonsearching support, like the name implies, characterizes support that is provided to someone who does not ask for it. A concerned parent preparing a snack for their child studying for an exam is one example, as we might infer from Vuong's account.

Nonsearching happens selectively in Western cultures, like when people nominate their unemployed friends for jobs knowing that they need the help even if they do not ask for it outright (Trimble & Kmec, 2011). In East Asian cultures, nonsearching may happen more frequently due to the norms that Vuong points out and it might also be broader in the types of support that flow through networks. Given how tightknit families are in East Asian cultures, this opens up the provision of new kinds of support that might otherwise be sanctioned in Western cultures. Welfare is a good example. Tightknit families in East Asian cultures are more likely to give monetary assistance to other family members and permit children to stay with their families well into adulthood, even when help-receivers do not ask for such help (Frankenberg et al., 2002).

In East Asian cultures, moving out of the family household does not hold the same gravity as it does in Western cultures, where it is touted as a rite of passage into adulthood and independence; by contrast, tightknit East Asian families insist instead on the nuclear family model, where multiple generations of family members live under the same roof. Put together, these arrangements offer some reprieve from financial burdens and their resultant stress that people face.

The Limits of Embeddedness: Differential Access to Social Support

As good as embeddedness is for social support in East Asian cultures, there are important limits created by some of those cultural beliefs as well. If we recall from Chapter 2, there is a latent patriarchy behind the expectations imposed upon women in East Asian cultures. Women are expected to be more subservient, kinder, and more emotional, echoes of a housewife ideal like what sociologists have observed in North America. Men, by contrast, are valorized as superior in general (Bian & Ikeda, 2018; Hofstede, 1991).

The patriarchy in East Asian cultural beliefs has repercussions on how people exchange social support and build their networks, all of which become gendered and unequal. To illustrate, I observe strong patterns of segregation between men's networks and women's networks. When examining how many of people's close friends are the same sex in Japan, I find that 63% of women have close friends who are all women and 35% of women have close friends who consist of some women. I also find that 49% of men have close friends who are exclusively men and 48% of men have close friends who consist of some men. The numbers show that men and women tend to form networks that are separated from one another.

In network science, this is called homophily, or the propensity to network with people who are similar to you in some way. More specifically, this is essentially gender homophily, networking between people who identify as the same gender. Gender homophily complicates social support and stress because networks that are homophilous are notoriously sticky and internally cohesive (Smith et al., 2014). They are very selective about who can get into the network and who can make the most of it. Put differently, the gendered segregation of networks also means that men's and women's networks are not very porous; they are accessible only to people of the same gender. Men's networks are accessible mostly to men, and likewise for women.

As a result of this network segregation, the types of stressors that men and women experience may vary greatly, as do their ability to procure social support. For one, the network segregation we observe compounds a status segregation between men and women. In the 2012 Japanese General Social Survey, when asked whether they believed it was important for a wife to help her husband's career than to have one herself, 43% of respondents completely or somewhat agreed, and 45% completely or somewhat disagreed.

This captures a core issue facing women in East Asia: they face more work-related stress from their networks and have fewer connections to help assuage such stressors. Men themselves and their networks typically have higher statuses and command greater workplace resources, including professional affiliations, clout, and information, than do women (Bian & Ikeda, 2018; Ikeda, 2012). This produces an inequality in the amount of labor women have to put in compared to men, such that women consistently work longer hours and for lower pay than their male counterparts at every level of education across every East Asian nation (Ko & Kim, 2018; Liu et al., 2018; Nemoto, 2013).

Combined with greater demands for housework, women are consistently relegated to inferior, often lower-paying roles than men in the workplace and to caregiver roles in the household. Women thus come to be predisposed to higher levels of work-related stress, job precarity, and have fewer instrumental means to resolve these issues (Jung et al., 2021; Won, 2016). These patriarchal social structures are so powerful that women tend to rely on their husbands to access the resources they need, including power, work opportunities, and information (Bian & Ikeda, 2018; Ikeda, 2012).

By the same token, however, the caregiving roles that women are permitted and socialized into lend well for their ability to build ties and grow their networks in general. Continuing with the example of Japan, there is a stark difference in the number of close friends reported between men versus women (Figure 4.2).

Most men and women report having "3 to 4" or "5 to 9" close friends, but men have noticeably fewer close friends than women on average, at best coming close to rival women on the number of close friends toward the upper end. More men also report having no close friends

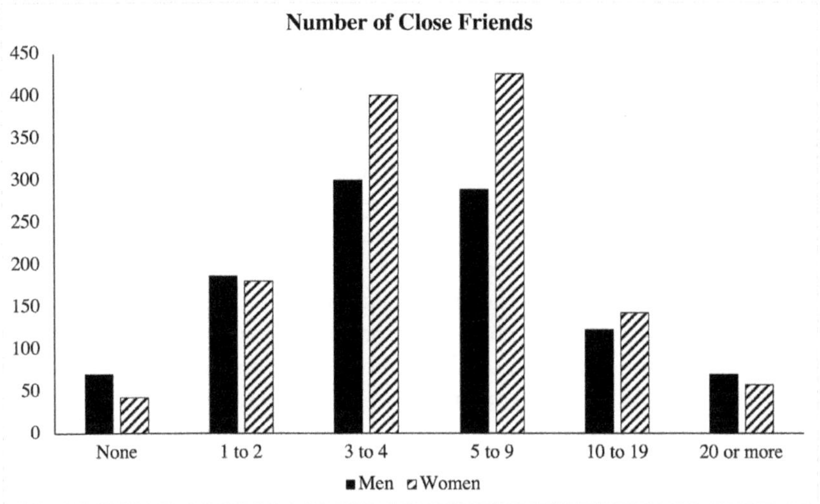

Figure 4.2 Number of close friends among men and women in Japan.

Source: Author's calculations using 2012 Japanese General Social Survey data from JGSS Research Center, Osaka University of Commerce, Japan (2016)

at all compared to women. Analyses of past versions of the Japanese General Social Survey show the same picture. From the 2003 version, for instance, Ikeda (2012) finds that women have 20% more ties to discuss important matters with than men.

A rich vein of network science tells us that having a larger network is on the whole a good thing for social support. In this case, East Asian women benefit from their larger network sizes because they gain access to a diversity of ties, have greater chances of getting support, and have greater likelihood of finding a good "match" for whatever needs they have in circumstances beyond the workplace (Au, 2019; Plickert et al., 2007; Wang, 2016).

A cross-comparative study of South Korean and Japanese workers over time reveals a more striking picture, that men not only derive most of their connections from the workplace, but these connections are more likely to fade out into retirement than those of women (Takahashi et al., 2020). These differences surface in later life when older men experience greater feelings of isolation, worse mental health, and worse ability to cope with stress than their female counterparts – a problem that has been exacerbated by the COVID-19 pandemic that sent cities shuttering down and beset residents with strict lockdown and social distancing guidelines (Sugaya et al., 2021; Wang, 2016).

Thus, although men might have more opportunities for upward mobility from their networks, they face cultural barriers to their ability to express themselves that results in smaller networks less ready to provide support. In the case of Japan (through the 2012 General Social Survey), we observe as much in a demographic rift in who seeks help. When prompted to consider who they sought help from the last time they experienced emotional or psychological problems, about 84% of women who responded chose someone to seek help from and just under 8% elected not to seek help. For men who responded, the numbers were vastly different, where only 70% of men who responded sought help and 17% elected not to seek any help from anyone when faced with psychological problems, nearly double the rate seen for women.

This is exacerbated by the instrumentality that defines a lot of the networking in East Asian cultures, especially for men who make most of their ties in the workplace. Men have even less cultural permission to ask for emotional kinds of help from their ties, since they were former colleagues (who, again, subsequently fade out when they venture into retirement). The inequality of social support we see in the gender divide reflects the entrenchment of cultural beliefs that stigmatize mental health and complicate the exchange of resources to alleviate the burden of stress; it is thus that the problems of stress and lack of support extend to identities that are sanctioned by East Asian cultures, like mental health patients themselves who are stigmatized, as touched upon in Chapter 3 and, as Chapter 5 will elaborate, become internalized in patients and professionals alike.

References

Alsubaie, M. M., Stain, H. J., Webster, L. A. D., & Wadman, R. (2019). The role of sources of social support on depression and quality of life for university students. *International Journal of Adolescence and Youth*, *24*(4), 484–496.

Au, A. (2019). The embodiment of social capital at individual and communal levels: Action, rewards, inequality, and new directions. *International Journal of Sociology and Social Policy*, *39*(9/10), 812–830.

Bian, Y. (1997). Bringing strong ties back in: Indirect ties, network bridges, and job searches in China. *American Sociological Review*, *62*(3), 366–385.

Bian, Y., & Ikeda, K. (2018). East Asian social networks. In R. Alhajj & J. Rokne (Eds.), *Encyclopedia of social network analysis and mining* (2nd ed., pp. 1–22). New York: Springer.

Brody, L. R., & Hall, J. A. (2010). Gender, emotion, and socialization. In J. C. Chrisler & D. R. McCreary (Eds.), *Handbook of gender research in psychology* (pp. 429–454). New York: Springer.

Brown, S. L., Nesse, R. M., Vinokur, A. D., & Smith, D. M. (2003). Providing social support may be more beneficial than receiving it: Results from a prospective study of mortality. *Psychological Science*, *14*(4), 320–327.

Chrostek, A., Grygiel, P., Anczewska, M., Wciórka, J., & Świtaj, P. (2016). The intensity and correlates of the feelings of loneliness in people with psychosis. *Comprehensive Psychiatry*, *70*, 190–199.

Cong, Z., & Silverstein, M. (2011). Intergenerational exchange between parents and migrant and non-migrant sons in rural China. *Journal of Marriage and Family*, *73*, 93–104.

Crohan, S. E., & Antonucci, T. C. (1989). Friends as a source of social support in old age. In R. G. Adams & R. Blieszner (Eds.), *Older adult friendship: Structure and process* (pp. 129–146). New York: SAGE.

Dour, H. J., Wiley, J. F., Roy-Byrne, P., Stein, M. B., Sullivan, G., Sherbourne, C. D., Bystritsky, A., Rose, R. D., & Craske, M. G. (2014). Perceived social support mediates anxiety and depressive symptom changes following primary care intervention. *Depression and Anxiety*, *31*(5), 436–442.

English Standard Version Bible. (2001). *ESV online*. Wheaton, IL: Crossway Bibles, Good News Publisher. Retrieved from https://esv.literalword.com/

Fei, X. (1992). *From the soil*. Thousand Oaks, CA: University of California Press. (Original work published 1947)

Frankenberg, E., Lillard, L., & Willis, R. J. (2002). Patterns of intergenerational transfers in Southeast Asia. *Journal of Marriage and Family*, *64*(3), 627–641.

Herbst-Damm, K. L., & Kulik, J. A. (2005). Volunteer support, marital status, and the survival times of terminally ill patients. *Health Psychology*, *24*, 225–229.

Hofstede, G. (1991). Empirical models of cultural differences. In N. Bleichrodt & P. J. D. Drenth (Eds.), *Contemporary issues in cross-cultural psychology* (pp. 4–20). Amsterdam: Swets & Zeitlinger Publishers.

House, J. S., Landis, K. R., & Umberson, D. (1988). Social relationships and health. *Science*, *241*, 540–545.

Ikeda, K. (2012). Differential effect of multiple social networks on public participation in Japan. In A. Daniere & H. Van Luong (Eds.), *The dynamics of social capital and civic engagement in Asia: Vibrant societies* (pp. 54–80). London: Routledge.

JGSS Research Center, Osaka University of Commerce, Japan. (2016). *Japanese General Social Survey 2012 (JGSS 2012)* [ZA6427 Data file Version 2.0.0]. Cologne: GESIS Data Archive. https://doi.org/10.4232/1.12604. Retrieved from https://search.gesis.org/research_data/ZA6427

Jung, J., Lippényi, Z., & Mun, E. (2021). Workplace volatility and gender inequality: A comparison of the Netherlands and South Korea. *Socio-Economic Review*, mwab026. https://doi.org/10.1093/ser/mwab026

Ko, E. J., & Kim, S. S. (2018). Intention to use flexible work arrangements: The case of workers in Korea and gender differences in motivation. *Journal of Organizational Change Management*, *31*(7), 1438–1460.

Kuiper, J. S., Zuidersma, M., Zuidema, S. U., Burgerhof, J. G., Stolk, R. P., Oude Voshaar, R. C., & Smidt, N. (2016). Social relationships and cognitive decline: A systematic review and meta-analysis of longitudinal cohort studies. *International Journal of Epidemiology*, *45*(4), 1169–1206.

Lin, N. (2001a). *Social capital: A theory of social structure and action*. Cambridge, MA: Cambridge University Press.

Lin, N. (2001b). Building a network theory of social capital. In N. Lin, K. Cook, & R. Burt (Eds.), *Social capital: Theory and research* (pp. 3–30). New York: Aldine de Gruyter.

Liu, L., MacPhail, F., & Dong, X. Y. (2018). Gender, work burden, and mental health in post-reform China. *Feminist Economics*, *24*(2), 194–217.

MacDonald, M. (2007). Social support for centenarians' health, psychological well-being, and longevity. *Annual Review of Gerontology and Geriatrics*, *27*(1), 107–127.

Miller, R. J., & Darlington, Y. (2002). Who supports? The providers of social support to dual-parent families caring for young children. *Journal of Community Psychology*, *30*(5), 461–473.

Nauck, B., & Arránz Becker, O. (2013). Institutional regulations and the kinship solidarity of women – results from 13 areas in Asia, Africa, Europe, and North America. *European Sociological Review*, *29*(3), 580–592.

Nemoto, K. (2013). Long working hours and the corporate gender divide in Japan. *Gender, Work & Organization*, *20*(5), 512–527.

Penwell, L. M., & Larkin, K. T. (2010). Social support and risk for cardiovascular disease and cancer: A qualitative review examining the role of inflammatory processes. *Health Psychology Review*, *4*(1), 42–55.

Piolatto, M., Bianchi, F., Rota, M., Marengoni, A., Akbaritabar, A., & Squazzoni, F. (2022). The effect of social relationships on cognitive decline in older adults: An updated systematic review and meta-analysis of longitudinal cohort studies. *BMC Public Health*, *22*(1), 1–14.

Plickert, G., Côté, R. R., & Wellman, B. (2007). It's not who you know, it's how you know them: Who exchanges what with whom? *Social Networks*, *29*(3), 405–429.

Schacter, H. L., & Margolin, G. (2019). The interplay of friends and parents in adolescents' daily lives: Towards a dynamic view of social support. *Social Development*, *28*(3), 708–724.

Schnall, S., Roper, J., & Fessler, D. M. (2010). Elevation leads to altruistic behavior. *Psychological Science*, *21*(3), 315–320.

Smith, J. A., McPherson, M., & Smith-Lovin, L. (2014). Social distance in the United States: Sex, race, religion, age, and education homophily among confidants, 1985 to 2004. *American Sociological Review*, *79*(3), 432–456.

Sugaya, N., Yamamoto, T., Suzuki, N., & Uchiumi, C. (2021). Social isolation and its psychosocial factors in mild lockdown for the COVID-19 pandemic: A cross-sectional survey of the Japanese population. *BMJ Open*, *11*(7), e048380.

Takahashi, S., Jang, S. N., Kino, S., & Kawachi, I. (2020). Gender inequalities in poor self-rated health: Cross-national comparison of South Korea and Japan. *Social Science & Medicine*, *252*, 112919.

Taylor, S. E. (2011). Social support: A review. In H. Friedman (Ed.), *The Oxford handbook of health psychology* (pp. 192–217). Oxford: Oxford University Press.

Tengku Mohd, T. A. M., Yunus, R. M., Hairi, F., Hairi, N. N., & Choo, W. Y. (2019). Social support and depression among community dwelling older adults in Asia: A systematic review. *BMJ Open*, *9*(7), e026667.

Thoits, P. A. (1995). Stress, coping and social support processes: Where are we? What next? *Journal of Health and Social Behavior*, *35*, 53–79.

Trimble, L. B., & Kmec, J. A. (2011). The role of social networks in getting a job. *Sociology Compass*, *5*(2), 165–178.

Tsai, Y. F., Yeh, S. H., & Tsai, H. H. (2005). Prevalence and risk factors for depressive symptoms among community-dwelling elders in Taiwan. *International Journal of Geriatric Psychiatry: A Journal of the Psychiatry of Late Life and Allied Sciences*, *20*(11), 1097–1102.

Uehara, E. S. (1990). Dual exchange theory, social networks, and informal social support. *American Journal of Sociology*, *96*(3), 521–557.

Uehara, E. S. (1995). Reciprocity reconsidered: Gouldner's moral norm of reciprocity and social support. *Journal of Social and Personal Relationships*, *12*(4), 483–502.

VanKim, N. A., & Nelson, T. F. (2013). Vigorous physical activity, mental health, perceived stress, and socializing among college students. *American Journal of Health Promotion*, *28*(1), 7–15.

Vuong, O. (2019, December 25). Ocean Vuong on war, sexuality and Asian-American identity | Amanpour and Company. *YouTube*. Retrieved from www.youtube.com/watch?v=9OZIwsk9cAM&t=586s&ab_channel=AmanpourandCompany

Wang, J., Mann, F., Lloyd-Evans, B., Ma, R., & Johnson, S. (2018). Associations between loneliness and perceived social support and outcomes of mental health problems: A systematic review. *BMC Psychiatry*, *18*(1), 1–16.

Wang, X. (2016). Subjective well-being associated with size of social network and social support of elderly. *Journal of Health Psychology*, *21*(6), 1037–1042.

Wellman, B., & Frank, K. (2001). Network capital in a multilevel world: Getting support from personal communities. In N. Lin, K. Cook, & R. S. Burt (Eds.), *Social capital: Theory and research* (pp. 233–273). New York: Aldine de Gruyter.

Wellman, B., & Wortley, S. (1990). Different strokes from different folks: Community ties and social support. *American Journal of Sociology*, *96*(3), 558–588.

Wills, T. A. (1991). Social support and interpersonal relationships. In M. S. Clark (Ed.), *Prosocial behavior* (pp. 265–289). Newbury Park, CA: SAGE.

Won, S. Y. (2016). State policy? Traditional gender stereotypes? Relative contributions of factors affecting positive work – family interface for working mothers in Korea. *Gender, Work & Organization*, *23*(2), 147–164.

Yang, Y. C., Boen, C., Gerken, K., Li, T., Schorpp, K., & Harris, K. M. (2016). Social relationships and physiological determinants of longevity across the human life span. *Proceedings of the National Academy of Sciences*, *113*(3), 578–583.

Yang, Y. C., McClintock, M. K., Kozloski, M., & Li, T. (2013). Social isolation and adult mortality: The role of chronic inflammation and sex differences. *Journal of Health and Social Behavior*, *54*(2), 183–203.

5 Cultural Beliefs and Professional Services

Professionals, Clinics, and Social Spaces

Clinics are commonly thought of as sterile physical spaces where doctors meet their patients. The prototypical patient enters the domain of the professional doctor in a state of *tabula rasa*, a blank slate, with nothing else but the suffering they carry from physiological ailments. There, they await solutions for their ailments meted out by the steady hand of a doctor.

A cultural and sociological perspective of social relations informs us that this is a rather oversimplified vision of reality that does not reflect reality. No actor walks free from preconceptions, biases, and values about *meaning* that are developed over a lifetime, programmed into them by the assent of fellow members of their culture. Chapter 2 outlined the architecture of values in East Asian cultures and Chapter 3 examined how it holds fast. This chapter examines how these conceptions dictate decisions made about the professional provision and receipt of services.

We might then begin by reconceptualizing the clinic itself. We could gain new insight into the dynamics that occur within clinics if we theorize them instead as social spaces. Social spaces are not merely physical spaces but cultural milieu replete with symbols that take on different meanings when patients and doctors alike bring their cultural beliefs into contact with one another.

Sociologists have offered prominent theories of social spaces. Eminent sociologist Andrew Abbott conceives of social spaces as "a system of actors in a set of locations" (2005, p. 246). In a nod to Georg Simmel's understanding of social structure, Sida Liu (2021) goes on to characterize social spaces in terms of the conformity and opposition within them, which offers a useful way to understand relations between spaces. I theorize clinics as social spaces in the sense that cultural beliefs are imported into them through actors, like doctors and patients, after which they actively shape the interactions between them. Like Liu's theory (2021), these interactions can involve how much actors agree or disagree with

DOI:10.4324/9781003308720-5

each other. But of core focus in my cultural view of social space is the structuration of provision of treatment by doctors and pursuit or receipt of treatment by patients that happens when their cultural beliefs come into contact with one another.

The design of spaces influences the social practices and outcomes within it when cultural beliefs interweave with the organization of space to impress upon actors within the space a sense of *order* and regularity, which they submit to (Loughran, 2016; Rawson, 2010). We can think here of Elijah Anderson's ethnography of low-income Black men and women surviving in the space of "the streets" of Philadelphia in heavily policed, low-class neighborhoods. Despite their less-than-ideal surroundings, these men and women's lives were affected not through the material conditions of dilapidation of their space but through the cultural beliefs that had come to inhabit it – something Anderson calls the "code of the street," which was "not the goal of product of any individual's actions but . . . the fabric of everyday life, a vivid and pressing milieu within which all local residents must shape their personal routines, [practices and] . . . relations" (Anderson, 2001, p. 326).

As this chapter will show, cultural beliefs come to structurally inform the ways that meanings of health, illness, and even medical history come to life through the interpretive processes behind the creation of meaning, namely, the indication and representation of things acted toward and the communication of self that establishes the importance of these representations (Au, 2017; Blumer, 1969).

The Embeddedness of Cultural Beliefs

Cultural Beliefs in Professional Practice

It is known that a physician is held to a higher standard of behavior by licensing boards, tasked to build trust and rapport with patients in their efforts to heal and save lives. Yet, professionals are no more immune to the cultural forces that sweep through society than the patients they serve. They, too, bring baggage to the table.

Through several case studies of East Asian doctor-patient relationships that I have analyzed over the years, I observed that it might be valuable for a doctor with continuity and knowledge about personal medical history, but that this is a double-edged sword. Highly influential for health and treatment outcomes, trust is an important part of the healing process, and takes a long time to build. But trust is also what slowly gives rise to unforeseen assumptions that might evoke conservative cultural sentiments and ultimately force patients to censor themselves.

In several case studies on physician-patient conflicts in Chinese communities, I found that physicians who were the most likely to be trusted on a personal level by their patients were those who knew their patients for the longest. Over time, physicians grew comfortable with their patients, building a relationship with them and assuming a kind of guardianship over their health. Yet, this also invited physicians to let loose their personal cultural beliefs – and judgments – in their communications with patients.

This is true of public medicine. In one case, Dr. Chang was a general practitioner in his privately owned, but publicly funded clinic, and had known his patients for decades. At a regular health checkup with one of them, when it came time to speak about sexual history and activity, Dr. Chang broke from the usual questions. Rather than asking, "what sexual activity have you had?" or something along those lines, Dr. Chang went on to ask about whether his patient "had a girlfriend." After his patient declined, Dr. Chang then noted that "he didn't have any sexual activity, then."

There are several assumptions emergent from Dr. Chang's cultural beliefs that distorted his communications with his patient. For one, the patient had turned out to be a sexual minority, and so understandably did not have a girlfriend. Second, Dr. Chang had assumed that sexual activity only transpired within the confines of a relationship. These two assumptions owe to traditional cultural beliefs about sexuality and relationships in East Asian cultures, normalizing heterosexuality and precluding all other sexual orientations. These assumptions stifled the patient's willingness to openly communicate stressors with Dr. Chang, quickly foreclosing the opportunity to venture into sexual and mental health discussions to do with his positionality.

In another case, Dr. Kim was a practicing general physician in a community clinic and had known his patients for years also. Once, a teenage girl entered his office in the middle of her second trimester. There, the girl sought advice about everyday stressors during a teenage pregnancy but responded to Dr. Kim's comments with what he later called a nonchalant attitude. Angered by her apparent apathy, Dr. Kim unleashed a tirade of comments about how he felt she was being too careless, having been pregnant to begin with, and even now after being so far along in the pregnancy. He went on to dismiss her pregnancy as a poor decision that would close opportunities for the rest of her life, radically shifting it into a different, less successful path that she had apparently been too immature to see. So forceful was his ire that he even went so far as to post the encounter on his personal social media accounts.

Like Dr. Chang, Dr. Kim's responses invoked East Asian cultural beliefs – about the role of children and educational success. As Chapter 2 described, children are burdened with stringent expectations about academic achievement, couched in views of education as the ultimate duty of a child and as a lifelong path to upward mobility both for the child and for their family. Deviance from these expectations, as we observe with Dr. Kim's account, is met with cultural sanctions and disapproval.

In these two vivid cases, we observe the cultural baggage that doctors bring to the clinic, lurking thinly beneath the veneer of professional identity. When opportunities to draw closer with patients arise, as they naturally do with physician-patient relationships, so too does the risk of inviting these cultural beliefs into patient communications – and behavioral expectations.

This is true of private medicine as well, which even more easily slips away from focusing on patient well-being. In an ethnography of health clinics in South Korea, I found much of the discourse that professionals used in patient discussions were designed to capitalize on experiences of mental health. In a telling example, Dr. Jeon, a doctor in the international clinic at a university health service, saw a patient who entered with a minor headache. There, the patient laid upon Dr. Jeon a whole roster of hypotheses about their own conditions drawn from WebMD: parasitic infections, meningitis, neurodegenerative diseases. Rather than addressing the symptoms as they were, Dr. Jeon referred the patient to a list of procedures just as long as the patient's list of hypotheses, he and encouraged the patient to speak up about any other "theories" that they might have, so as to test them as well. The distress and anxiety clearly bubbling over in the patient went unchecked by Dr. Jeon.

Other physicians often followed suit. Physicians entertained the wildest theories that patients had about their health trawled from the internet, coming to recommend a whole gamut of expensive and time-consuming procedures that magnified patient anxiety. Though one may chalk this up to the nature of privatized medicine and the incentive to sell, the way through which these procedures were marketed openly manipulated patient insecurities and spoke powerfully about the cultural dearth of consciousness about mental health itself among professionals in the region.

Such influences that cultural beliefs have over the way doctors think, practice, and interact with patients speak to the subject of power that emerges within clinics as social spaces. Cultural beliefs transform innocuous physiological symptoms and expectations of behavior into matters of conformity or deviance, speaking to the embeddedness of meanings in spaces (Lamont, 2000). The extent to which patient medical histories and profiles align with the values outlined by cultural beliefs, such as about heteronormativity or about educational achievement, determines how doctors make patients feel about themselves. As symbolic interactionists classically note, meaning is created with two kinds of interpretive processes: (1) indicating the representations of things that we are acting toward and (2) communicating the self in ways that establish the importance of these representations (Blumer, 1969).

In both public and private medicine, doctors inadvertently make gestures toward cultural beliefs in their communication with patients. As they do, they signal to patients a moral rubric with which to evaluate their own medical history and decisions. Centering the meanings of personal medical history and decisions around the doctor's underlying cultural beliefs strips the patient of agency and plants a new kind of professional power within the doctor, coming to direct people's activities in relation to them (Simmel, 1990/1997, p. 237; Dennis & Martin, 2005).

A 2016 large-scale survey of medical students in the United States, Brazil, Ghana, Nigeria, and China investigated this kind of professional bias. The results were striking. They revealed that among the five countries, medical students in China had the lowest social and policy acceptance of mental illnesses. Chinese professionals are mired in cultural beliefs about mental illnesses, stigmatized as defections of character and predispositions toward violence (Stefanovics et al., 2016).

These differences were corroborated in subsequent surveys at medical schools in China (Zhu et al., 2018). Using interviews with medical professionals in the region, Luo and colleagues (2018) observed that physicians commonly felt that merely associating with mentally ill patients would make them lose "face," something they feared would depreciate their social standing within the profession and society in general. Indeed, we observe that the embeddedness of actors within dense East Asian networks additionally amplified the boons of face and the banes of stigma as individual achievements and failures reflected on familial honor. These rigidly held misconceptions of mental illness as defections of character or violent dispositions may thus come to shape even physician perceptions of mental illness.

This is further evinced by the hierarchy of statuses that exist among doctors by their fields. In East Asia, psychologists, psychiatrists, and doctors who treat mental health issues are perceived by their profession as belonging to a lower status (Zhu et al., 2018). That cultural beliefs about mental health are so engrained in the professional ecology holds significant repercussions for professional practice. Doctors may be blinded to the subject of mental health and neglect it as a legitimate ailment their patients face. Doctors may also dismiss patient concerns about mental health if brought up, failing to refer patients to appropriate mental health resources or even refusing to take patients who wish to seek out mental health resources for fear of losing professional status. Worse, if doctors are familiar with the patient's family (which is often the case with longer physician-patient relationships), they may inadvertently discuss their patients' mental illnesses with their family without explicit consent.

In theorizing the manifestations of cultural beliefs in professional malpractice, I do not mean to spotlight a deficiency in professional ethics but to magnify the power that doctors have and the added significance of addressing latent cultural beliefs that animate their professional judgments.

Professional Power and Patients

Cultural beliefs seize hold in patients as much as in their doctors. Doctors are professionals who wield a considerable amount of power within the clinic. They wield organizational command over the dynamics of a clinic, dispensing orders to other healthcare workers lower in the hierarchy. They command the patient's body as well, offering expertise that is at once personal and professional, rendering the body alien to the patient herself – transforming it from something that the patient thinks she knows to something that only the doctor does through scientific, esoteric procedures, diagnoses, terms, and treatments. In East Asia, doctors are professionals with also a significant amount of status in society at large.

Given these multiple sources of power, when doctors signal interpretive representations of what they expect to be proper behavior and life choices, they likely exert a hard-to-resist influence over patients to conform as well. This disincentivizes patients to be forthcoming about their stressors and mental health experiences. Moreover, the influence that doctors have over their patients may also be growing in an age of mass information.

In a recent survey experiment on a new tool to help minority patients decide on which new medication to take for their cholesterol (Hopkin et al., 2019), I found that they tended to be very indecisive about their decisions. The decision aid was an online ranking tool that helped patients decide between several different types of drugs, based on benefits and costs that were laid out by the tool. Patients could toggle what benefits and costs they cared most about, after which the tool would then "rank" the best matching drugs for their profile (Figure 5.1). My team and I tested how well the tool worked for a group of patients who had access to it (a treatment group) and another group who did not (a control group).

At the end of the study, we found that participants who did *not* have access to the decision aid had significantly higher decisional conflict, confusion, uncertainty than those who did. More than an isolated study of one particular type of drug, our study laid bare a deeper problem of misinformation and confusion – something prevalent among patients as they make mundane and critical health decisions, ultimately enhancing their susceptibility to the cultural beliefs and worldviews of figures of authority like doctors.

The imbalance in power between patients and doctors that leads patients to self-censor themselves is paradoxically enhanced by an age of mass information. Over the past decade, patients in healthcare models around the world have been afforded an increasing amount of choice and control over their own treatment courses.

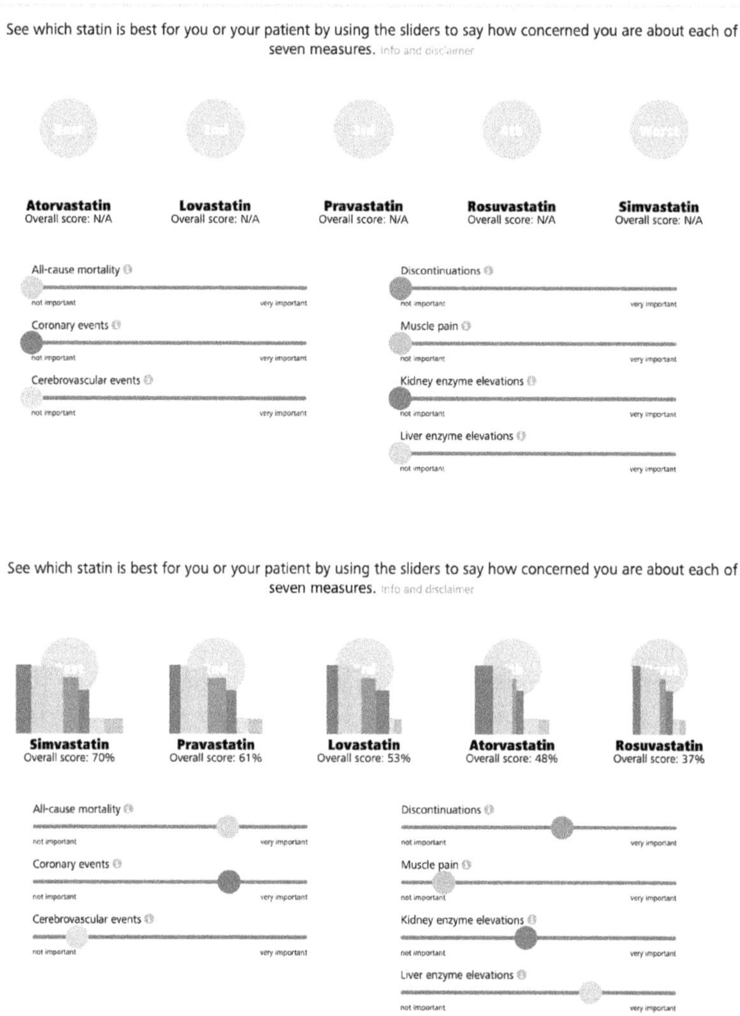

Figure 5.1 Exemplar online ranking tool for cholesterol drugs (statins). The top panel shows the default status of the tool. The bottom panel shows an example of its use, where users have selected their preferences and the tool has responded with a ranking of most appropriate drugs.

Source: Publicly available at http://lse.live.kiln.digital/statins/

Pressed to develop more sensitive treatment options shaped around the needs of the patient, greater initiatives have sprung up to balance the power dynamic and decision-making process between physicians and patients (Au, 2018, 2019; Dalma et al., 2020; Department of Health, 2000; Nimmon & Stenfors-Hayes, 2016; Stewart, 1995).

In response, however, there quickly arose too much choice and too much information. Citizenship scientists have sprung up like wildfire around the globe, particularly as preference for wellness begins to assert authority over burgeoning lifestyle, nutrition, and exercise programs (Naci & Ioannidis, 2015). Health experts such as Dr. Oz have sprung up and developed inroads into mass media outlets to vocalize paid opinions about a perpetual line-up of health products to push patients towards idealized standards of wellness and body image. Transforming medical care into health consumption represents an attempt to place as much health information as possible at the patient's disposal, and so empowers them by affording them greater control over their own health maintenance and outcomes (Baggott & Forster, 2008).

In theory, there are clear merits to this ethic. It potentially enriches patient-physician encounters by generating more productive conversations with patients who are better educated and prepared to table nuanced inquiries with greater prospects for developing actionable health strategies. In practice, however, there are important drawbacks, which we observed in the cases of physician-patient interactions that I presented earlier.

More than pushing patients toward more decisive action and collaboration about the health information they receive, the growth of health informatics in an age of mass information contributes to patient indecision and decisional conflict. Against the backdrop of an effort in social epidemiology, health psychology, and medicine to place more control of treatment plans in patients' own hands (Allsop et al., 2004; Baggott et al., 2014; Coulter, 1998; Linder et al., 2011; Nilsen et al., 2006; Or & Karsh, 2009), there are declines in patients' ability to decide effectively on a treatment option that are becoming more visible, and which place a significantly greater onus on doctors – who may thus be given greater liberty to let loose conservative cultural beliefs that influence their patients to do the same. Indeed, patients may feel compelled to accede to expectations that doctors convey per their cultural beliefs.

Patients are susceptible to cultural beliefs that devalue mental health when it is presented by doctors in East Asian cultures. But at the same time, they are just as susceptible to these cultural beliefs on their own. Put differently, being confronted by conservative cultural beliefs in a doctor may be doubly damaging given that patients themselves are often grappling with cultural demands from their families. This results in the historically low treatment patterns we observe in East Asia. Studies have found that just 20% of people with mental health disorders sought professional help in Japan and Korea, with the number falling to about 0.15% in China (Ishikawa et al., 2016; Nagar, 2022; Que et al., 2019).

In a similar vein, we have ample evidence of a growing systemic problem of misinformation. We observe as much in organizational settings, such as business organizations (Edmunds & Morris, 2000), workplace settings (Kirsch, 2000), and science (Bawden, 2001). We observe this also among healthcare practitioners, such as with professional perceptions of mental illnesses, particularly in East Asia (Hall & Walton, 2004). In fact, the World Health Organization has singled out mental health stigma as a pressing area for action, identifying mental illness as the most significant burden of disease in developed countries and predicting its costs would exceed that of cancer and cardiovascular disorders in the future (World Health Organization, 2008, 2019).

Toward Resolution

Enhancing Professional Sensitivity: Complexity and Reflexivity

The previous sections discussed the myriad ways that East Asian cultural beliefs about mental health seep into professional judgments of patient health and, by extension, how patients think about themselves ultimately. Rather than distancing culture from practice, I suggest the solution lies in foregrounding and developing cultural sensitivity in practice. The remainder of this chapter discusses two interrelated approaches to healthcare reform that aim to ultimately reduce mental health problems and improve mental health service use: culture-specific services and a complexity theory perspective that posits the need for self-organization on a systemic level obtained through local interactions.

The first approach focuses on working toward a balance of culture-specific and culture-general approaches (Benzanson & James, 2007). There is a vital need for researchers to understand the mental health of East Asians in recognition of social complexities that may differ from other cultural backgrounds and which call for greater attention to educational policies for specific cultures among healthcare practitioners. Some treatments have been developed, such as Buddhist theories in counseling or psychotherapy, but they require more investigation into efficacy and outcomes (Cheng & Tse, 2014).

For practitioners, this means being reflexive about their positionality, recognizing their own status as an outsider or insider to the cultures of their patients – and familiarity with the values of specific cultures in order to build therapeutic relationships that improve treatment progress through self-esteem and adherence (Wampold, 2001).

This also means recognizing the social conditions to which patients are subject. To illustrate, whatever social support the family provides is shaped by the very cultural norms embedded in its structure. Conversely, that family can aggravate mental health problems is because of these very norms as well. Social support from family members within East Asian families is received under the expectation of conformity to their cultural norms and assigned roles. Children experience more pressure to succeed in education for familial social status, and while this has been found to reduce their likelihood of developing externalizing problems, it also reduces the efficacy of mastery – the individual perception of ability to handle stress – for everyone in the family.

Thus, mastery and sense of control become eroded by obligations of complacency and submission to culturally assigned roles. Similarly, other mental health coping mechanisms can be ruled out by family norms. Changing the meaning of a situation, for example, is a common strategy but would not work in the context of immigration or sexual minorities, given their urgency and sense of trauma as stressors. Avoidance or detachment from family itself as a source of distress is also common, but would also fail, because of the importance of family in non-Western, collectivistic cultures.

Furthermore, discussing mental health problems themselves with family or seeking professional help within these cultures is highly discouraged because of stigma. Mental health disorders are perceived as curses to the family, rather than legitimate health issues, and emotional suppression is actually seen as maturity, rather than the mental health aggravator that it is.

Nevertheless, implicated in this approach is an appreciation for culture as a lens for understanding how individuals conceptualize mental illness (Bojuwoye, 2001). Since professional help is discouraged in East Asian cultures – due to the cultural stigma associated with mental health disorders, perceived as curses to the family, and the preference for emotional suppression – the assurance of diagnostic accuracy and appropriateness of treatments requires addressing cultural context (Pedersen, 1997; Tatman, 2004).

In a similar vein, a second approach calls upon complexity theory to conceptualize healthcare reform. Complexity theory figures around the model of an open, dynamic, adaptive system to be addressed holistically (Morrison, 2005), wherein individuals shape their environment to the effect of creating global level change from local-level interactions (Paley, 2010). Within health, applications of the theory have been found in palliative care (Munday et al., 2003), supply and demand of health care (Brailsworth et al., 2011), health education (Bleakley, 2010; Doll & Trueit, 2010), among other areas (see Litaker et al., 2006). Its distinction from the first approach relies on its conception of an interplay of events that is characterized by ambiguity or multiple ways of understanding over a single representation (Mennin, 2010a). Only in this way could the messiness and overlapping possibilities of lived experiences be accounted for, making it ideal for navigating the multi-faceted issues pertinent to mental health. Reluctance from East Asian patients to disclose feelings, for instance, may be rooted in a combination of cultural obligations – containing emotions to appease standards of maturity or fear of stigmatization from family.

Drawing from complexity theory, teaching reflexivity in health education (local interactions) would improve self-organization to the effect of creating a more efficient, adaptive, complex system (global patterns) that better addresses the plurality of cultural principles underlying mental health problems among East Asians.

A complexity theory perspective can be brought to the healthcare team as a unit of analysis to proffer insights on how to improve efficiency in clinical settings (Arrow & Henry, 2010). Scholars employing this theory conceive the team as a form of collective intelligence organized around collaboration and sharing knowledge. The clinical setting effectively becomes an open system perpetually regulating and adjusting through feedback spurred by experiences in changing environments. Thus, applied complexity theory focuses our attention on the ecology that shapes actions within them rather than just the thoughts of individual practitioners (Bleakley, 2010; Mennin, 2010a). Some scholars urge the need for introducing diversity to teams, where different skills, knowledge, and abilities are shared to facilitate self-organization and adaptive learning (Mennin, 2010a, 2010b).

Yet, this application of complexity theory has drawn criticism for its treatment of the connection between order and design (Paley, 2010). Studies have been accused of misinterpreting the idea of self-organization. Mennin's (2010b) conception, for instance, would depend on members of a team consciously gathering to plan and design effective treatment in preparation for and particular to individuals from certain cultures. Order and design in this scheme become causally linked, running counter to their apparent dissociation intended by original complexity theory (Paley, 2010). In keeping with a process where global structures are explained by local interactions between individual units and their immediate environments, a self-organizing system involves individuals acting unilaterally and blind to the phenomenon they might create (Paley, 2010).

What are the benefits of separating order and design? At first, it may appear to be a pointless theoretical abstraction with no bearing on clinical practice. However, inherent in this rebuttal is another assumption: that the clinical conditions required for each individual to perform efficaciously are already existent. That, after all, is the only way a global pattern could emerge through individual conduct without collaboration. The difficulty thereafter – glaringly apparent – is how to ascertain this standard of conduct. Cultural reflexivity lends itself as a critical element of this potential reform.

Reflexivity refers to the ability to engage with and understand how one's social locations have shaped their understanding of their world. It helps practitioners understand culture in the way it is lived, as well as the way it can be variable and contradictory across different circumstances (Aronowitz et al., 2015). In other words, it instills a consciousness that trains practitioners to appreciate layered meanings and multiple potential explanations for the emergence of a mental health issue in East Asians; when healthcare practitioners are capable of doing so individually, treatment also becomes more efficient by ruling out the need to rely on continual consultation with others and preserving the potential for self-organization.

The ways in which reflexivity can be obtained are fragmented. A recent systematic review found that literature does not support one educational technique to the exclusion of all others (Landy et al., 2016): methods of reflection, transcultural encounters, values awareness, disorienting situations, experiential learning, debriefing all managed to improve reflexivity. Although this indicates a paucity of research in charting the efficacy of each (type of) educational method for reflexivity, it demonstrates the versatility of reflexivity and makes available a greater number of options to reforming health education. Furthermore, it helps to satisfy the need for cultural sensitivity in health education and treatment in research and clinical environments.

To illustrate, individuals who experience multiple identity problems – such as being both an immigrant and a sexual minority –are, in fact, likely to experience even greater stress than those who experience either one. More importantly, however, is how such circumstances that anticipate mental health problems are *not* just compounded in terms of stress, but also *interact with each other*. Take the case of a depression patient who also identifies as a sexual minority immigrating from a collectivistic culture. In this case, while he/she might be thankful for family providing a much-needed social support function, he/she could also be clandestinely suppressed "in the closet" and distressed by their attitude toward sexual minorities. Consequently, fear of upsetting the status quo eventually grows to become a stressor itself; at the same time it prevents the honest communication and resolution of other stressors.

What recommendations can we garner from the complex nature of mental health and the family? (1) Physicians, practitioners, and officials should recognize the overlapping, accumulative nature of stigma across multiple dimensions – mental health, homosexuality – and their relationship with the family. Families are often contacted in the event of risky or self-harm behaviors with roots in mental health. Contacting family about such problems may often endanger an individual in East Asian cultures that repudiate the legitimacy of mental health, risking social isolation and disappointment. Greater efforts should be made to culturally sensitize officials to such circumstances and improve trust, confidentiality, and openness between practitioners and patients.

(2) In a similar vein, practitioners should be sensitized to the problems family could pose that patients *themselves* might be unable to recognize and design culture-specific ways of communicating about such issues and developing their solutions. For instance, urging individuals to *detach*

from family might normally be an adequate strategy but would be a terrible way of communicating this strategy, likely inviting rejection.

Similarly, advising people to reinterpret the situation might be impossible, in face of the potential stressors they might be experiencing or masking. What patients do not say is just as important as what they do: particularly in East Asian cultures, patients are accustomed to languages that draw upon metaphors and indirect, rather than direct, expressions of meaning. Practitioners should be aware of this circumstance and develop prompts to sufficiently tease out and identify problems that patients do not overtly report.

(3) Services should adopt a family-oriented approach or component. Existing services also overburden counseling with the individual, often charging them with the task of confrontation and confession should the need arise, in spite of the aforementioned complications that family-relations pose. Keeping this in mind, bringing family into particular sessions and addressing them *with* the patient in focus would be crucial for maximizing on long-term benefits – not only resolving individual problems but also ensuring families are more educated, sensitive, and responsive to the causes and circumstances of mental health problems.

(4) Mental health itself also deserves greater access and recognition. Its stigma extends from hostility, where they are imagined as curses, to defamation, in which they are not recognized as health problems. Greater resources should be invested in raising public awareness of the depths and complexities within mental health and its problems, as well as in the mental health treatment practice, counseling programs, and services to connect individuals to such practitioners. In this regard, costs should be lowered and its coverage made a part of existing health coverage or insurance programs.

Enhancing Patient Understanding: Online Decision Aids and Tools

How do we enhance cultural understandings of mental health for patients? Part of the issue, as this chapter has discussed, homes in on the cultural baggage that physicians bring to the table when discussing patient health. A solution for this thus requires us to tweak the conventional model of decision-making where one party takes the lead in decision-making, which is typically the physician. I propose that we make use of online decision aids for mental health. Decision aids are an affordable, accessible, and easily scalable tool for educating patients about mental health issues and their existing biases, leaving them more confident and empowered. What results is a greater propensity for patients to make healthcare decisions even of more drastic measures, such as seeking out mental health services (Willemsen et al., 2006).

This section provides a four-step guideline for the application of online decision aids in reducing patient indecision, such as their conceptualization, user experience design, efficacy testing, and implementation in broader settings.

1. *Conceptualizing Online Decision Aids*

There is a preexisting sense of uncertainty and decisional conflict among patients toward health decisions. Evidently, the mass amounts of information available to patients on the internet do not alleviate but potentially exacerbate the feelings of uncertainty and indecision they approach health problems and decisions with (Barry et al., 2011). What is critical is deciding *what* information should be actionized to best deal with their circumstances, mediated with other lifestyle and health concerns.

Being presented with excessive amounts of information has been linked to a psychological paradox of choice: where having more choice paradoxically creates less, not more, satisfaction, and, by extension, greater decisional conflict (Bennett et al., 2010; Schwartz et al., 2002; see also Speier et al., 1999). In physician-patient interactions, this decisional conflict has taken form in a general sense of uncertainty about how and the extent to which patient preferences should be integrated in practice (Fowler et al., 2011).

There is pressing need for information to be filtered and organized by professionals and sensitized to patients' particular lifestyle demands. Online decision aids may reduce decisional conflict and improve decisional self-efficacy and preparation for decision-making; patients also tend to make less variable and more beneficial choices compared to those who do not.

In my own experiment of an online decision aid for cholesterol drugs, I found that users who used the tool with moderate concerns for all adverse effects were more likely to rank simvastatin as first choice, pravastatin instead of atorvastatin as second choice, and atorvastatin as third choice. These decisions better responded to the fact that simvastatin and atorvastatin have greater benefits, whereas pravastatin has better tolerability and harm profile (Naci et al., 2013), compared to other statins.

How do we decide what to include in a decision aid? Theoretically, I propose an inductive approach. My team's online statin-ranking decision aid first identified an existing problem (cholesterol), and finally included five statins and seven adverse effects for patients to toggle in the tool after an extensive network meta-analysis. I similarly suggest that researchers must first decide (a) a given problem, (b) the treatment options available, and (c) their most consequential consequences and considerations for patients, by cross-examining vast bodies of preexisting studies with systematic reviews, meta-analyses, and complementary measurements of inconsistency, such as the I2.

Systematic reviews and meta-analyses help to evaluate the quality of evidence concerning a given treatment, showing clinically important effects of similar magnitude while testing for differences underpinning study results (heterogeneity) or whether variation in findings is due to chance alone (homogeneity) (Higgins et al., 2003). Furthermore, applying an I2 quantity complements these approaches by testing for the degree of *in*consistency between trials in studies and even across meta-analyses of different sizes, types of studies, and types of outcome data (ibid). These approaches should be the default for designing tools to improve indecision.

There are myriad boons for the decision aid informed by such an inductive approach. I note the success of my own decision aid, verified with our experiment, but also observe that it gains credence from a growing body of quasi-experimental research on decision aids that also corroborate their positive effect on patient satisfaction with decision-making (O'Connor, 1995; O'Connor et al., 2017; Stacey et al., 2017) and patient treatment adherence (O'Connor et al., 1999).

Moyo et al. (2018), for instance, conducted a meta-analysis to find that decision aids were conducive to improving smoking behaviors in general. Brunette et al. (2015) showed that two months after using their decision aid, a statistical increase was observed of 71% of respondents having tried to quit, and 11% to 47% successfully obtaining varying degrees of abstinence. Among those who continued smoking, there was similarly a statistically significant decrease from a daily mean of 18.1 to 12.8 cigarettes.

2. *User Experience-Informed Designs of Online Decision Aids*

User experience (UX) is a practice-oriented theory that sits on the interstices of ergonomics and human-computer interface with the overarching objective of creating user experiences both useful and desirable (Mullins, 2015, p. 1). UX has since gained prominence in the design of digital customer-facing applications of businesses, inspiring a roster of design ontologies, such as navigation and findability, and ways to achieve them in digital layouts, such as drop-down menus, bar menus, and swipe-based content blocks.

I propose that insights from UX are synergistic with the large and complex amounts of information that researchers must process in Step (1), enabling researchers to translate it into an accessible format for patients. The goal of online decision aids is to collaboratively allow users to make a health decision about a given health problem in a way that minimizes misinformation, decisional uncertainty, and decisional dissatisfaction.

I thus propose that the UX design of online decision aids begin with *minimalism*. This principle of lean design is especially suited for reducing patient confusion. Online decision aids ought to visually present the most compelling information in the least number of bytes: aids should only visually focus on the (a) given problem, (b) treatment options available, and (c) their most consequential consequences and considerations for patients identified in Step (1). This assures patients that the most important information they need to assess in making their health decision is that which is presented there, laying to rest patients' speculative theories from information overload on online sources like WebMD.

Having a trimmed menu of options for users as the default appearance of the tool improves the affective state of patient users when they use it, which has an important effect on how they make decisions (Zhou et al., 2014). The design of decision aids can accomplish this by reducing the amount of information present, as well as separating and hiding any meta-information that is only needed for prospective or less experienced patients.

This could include the definitions of common mental health illnesses, their adverse effects, and symptoms, which might be meta-information that only appears when patients click a certain button to reveal it.

I further propose that there be an interactive component for users to have voice in the decision-making process, but for this to be confined to the risk profiles and adverse effect concerns. I suggest that the online decision aid works most efficaciously at a higher-level ontology: that is, the decision aid most reduces decisional uncertainty and misinformation when used to decide among treatment options of the same category (e.g., comparing different anti-depressant drugs), not to decide among different treatment categories altogether (e.g., weighing anti-depressant drugs vs. exercise). Patients would thus be allowed to feed their personal medical history into the online decision aid by self-rating and weighing their degree of concern with the adverse effects from possible treatment options, such as users reporting the same level of concern for different kinds of adverse effects.

I finally propose that treatment options for a given mental health illness be calibrated and *ranked* based on patients' tolerance for how suitable each option is. A patient may rank their own concerns about adverse effects, such as inability to function, constipation from drug use, fear of being found out by their families, and so on after which the online decision aid would produce a ranking for the type of treatment options recommended – such as therapy first, psychiatry second, and anti-depressant drugs third, and so on.

Ranking symptoms, effects, and treatment options of mental health illnesses directly is an intuitive way to distill them into actionable decisions for patients. UX researchers Sparling and Sen (2011), for instance, observed a greater cognitive load associated with more granular rating systems, such as a 100-point slider, compared to less granular systems, like the direct ranking of treatment options that we propose. Users need not process any index, so much as know that one treatment option is simply better than the other. Gallego et al. (2013) have found similar results by comparing designs of Android apps, finding that a more parsimonious ranking of options like ours is more intuitive to users as a feedback method because it resonates with a popular paradigm of UX in the Social Web for rating, such as ratings of Amazon goods.

Indeed, other popular examples of large and complex amounts of information being condensed into ranking visualizations include Morningstar's popular equity rating system, which ranks public equities using a scale of five "stars." A "five-star" rating represents the most attractive opportunity (a company whose shares are priced at a steep discount to their intrinsic value) and a "one-star" rating represents the least attractive opportunity (a company whose shares are priced at an expensive premium to their intrinsic value). This simplified visualization has been found to reduce retail investors' uncertainty, improve their decisional satisfaction, and encourage them to make more informed and sustainable investment decisions (Blake & Morey, 2000). Similarly, I propose that more parsimonious rankings of treatment options on a relative scale in online decision aids allow for more informed health decisions by patients.

3. Testing Online Decision Aids

After designing online decision aids, I propose testing them prior to launch to screen their efficacy. There are two possible ways of doing so: pilot studies and the Delphi method. Experiments are one method for conducting a pilot study. They minimize bias through several mechanisms, such as to standardize intervention and introduce double blinding without going so far as to reinforce implementation by providers or participation by patients. Their ability to identify causality in direct effects, furthermore, is well recognized and lends well to assessing the efficacy of interventions such as online decision aids (Imai et al., 2013).

Singal et al. (2014) succinctly capture the boons of experimental designs in their remarks that

> there are no requirements regarding provider expertise, and equipment quality may be variable. Similarly, providers are not restricted in terms of offering concurrent therapies or crossing over patients on-and-off therapy, which can lead to higher rates of drug – drug interactions and make it less clear if any effect was truly related to the intervention of interest.
>
> (p. e45)

Furthermore, randomized control trials remove barriers to access, such as providing the decision aid test for free, removing the need to be referred by a professional, and eliminating the need for patient acceptance and adherence over extended periods of time (ibid.; Flay et al., 2005; Sanson-Fisher et al., 2007).

An alternative expedited method of testing online decision aids is the Delphi method. The general premise of the Delphi method consists of polling a panel of experts for their opinions on a question, issuing them controlled feedback regarding such opinions, and repolling to allow them to respond to input from other panel members (Adler & Ziglio, 1996; Landeta, 2006; de Meyrick, 2003). Given that for many health issues there exists an appropriate body of knowledge possessed by a group of recognized experts (de Meyrick, 2003), the Delphi method is particularly useful for honing the impact of online decision aids and the precision of the health information they communicate.

4. *Areas of Implementation for Online Decision Aids*

I home in on two areas of implementation for online decision aids: clinics and policy.

At a clinical level, online decision aids offer physicians and patients the ability to visualize the most prevalent concerns powerfully and succinctly for possible treatment options. Online decision aids would thus enhance physician-patient consultations by improving patients' mental health literacy and orienting both parties to the same expectations in pursuing a course of action.

Dev and colleagues (2019) conducted a qualitative study of postpartum women and find that women valued decision aids because they

> enhanced their understanding of benefits and potential side effects of contraceptive methods, and *dispel contraceptive myths*; this led to a feeling of empowerment to make informed decisions . . . [and] set realistic expectations about potential side effects and maintaining confidentiality.
>
> (pp. 4, 8, italics added)

We observe here the merits of online decision aids for dispelling myths about mental health the same way Dev's decision aids reduced contraceptive myths for postpartum women. Just as important, we observe the significance of online decision aids as informative references for patients *and physicians* as a source of medical information (De Leo et al., 2006). The web interactive format of online decision aids makes them further accessible and equitable additionally because their use does not involve costs or physician recommendations.

At a policy level, online decision aids can improve the collaborative efforts that comprise the policymaking process, and have ample room to be implemented at a wider level through policy.

For one, online decision aids can involve policymakers by consulting them in Step (4) testing of the online decision aid through the Delphi Method, during which policymakers may act as experts who offer their opinions about how feasible and useful the decision aid is (Tso et al., 2011, p. 4).

Second, online decision aids can inform policymakers located in relevant governing authorities, such as physician and medical associations and governmental health departments, of the state of medical problems at any given time by providing up-to-date visualizations of the most pressing patient concerns and, by extension, health priorities. Oliver et al. (2017), for instance, identify using network data that UK health policymakers' sources of information are less so government websites or directors of public health but more personal contacts who tended to be mid-level managers in the National Health Service with alarmingly no direct expertise in public health.

Online decision aids could thus serve as an important source of medical expertise for consultation by policymakers, distilling comprehensive research evidence to inform and support policy decisions. Given that there is already substantial interest in participatory research, demonstrated by broad media coverage of health-related behaviors, which could be leveraged to facilitate recruitment for pilot studies. And with health consciousness at an all-time high, there is evidently an audience keenly interested in health and wellness to welcome the increased use of online decision aids.

Ultimately, there remains a growing problem of patient and physician misinformation borne of cultural beliefs and growing volumes of information exchanged on online communication platforms that have accelerated informational diffusion at the expense of quality control (Bawden & Robinson, 2009; Eppler & Mengis, 2004; Eysenbach & Jadad, 2001; McMullan, 2006).

Digital media platforms have intensified the diffusion of information through social exchanges in groups, forums, pages, and posts, evinced by how users increasingly cite them as sources of real information distinct from, and at times even more valuable than, traditional media news outlets (Au & Chew, 2017). The sheer availability of information online has aggravated the problem of misinformation when it comes to mental health, lending to ill-conceived attempts to manage one's own health care independently.

As a result, there is much room for professionals and patients like to improve their understanding of mental health issues and their personal cultural beliefs that inhibit this within East Asian cultures. Remedying this issue requires healthcare reform, with professional reflexivity playing a key role in the process, as well as superior education for alleviating East Asian cultural biases toward mental health for professionals and patients alike through easily accessible public education tools like online decision aids.

References

Abbott, A. (2005). Linked ecologies. *Sociological Theory*, *23*, 245–274.

Adler, M., & Ziglio, E. (1996). *Gazing into the oracle: The Delphi method and its application to social policy and public health*. London: Jessica Kingsley Publishers.

Allsop, J., Jones, K., & Baggott, R. (2004). Health consumer groups in the UK: A new social movement? *Sociology of Health & Illness*, *26*(6), 737–756.

Anderson, E. (2001). *Code of the street: Decency, violence, and the moral life of the inner city*. New York: W. W. Norton & Company.

Aronowitz, R. Deener, A., Keene, D., Schnittker, J., & Tach, L. (2015). Cultural reflexivity in health research and practice. *American Journal of Public Health*, *105*, 403–408.

Arrow, H., & Henry, K. B. (2010). Using complexity to promote group learning in health care. *Journal of Evaluation in Clinical Practice*, *16*, 861–866.

Au, A. (2018). Online physicians, offline patients: Professional identity and ethics in social media use. *International Journal of Sociology and Social Policy*, *38*(5/6), 474–483.

Au, A. (2019). Why physician guidance matters: A night of neuralgia, meningitis, and WebMD. *The Annals of Family Medicine*, *17*(5), 462–464.

Au, A., & Chew, M. (2017). Managing emotional reaction, conveyance, and detachment on Facebook and Instagram. *Bulletin of Science, Technology, & Society*, *37*(3), 127–137.

Baggott, R., Allsop, J., & Jones, K. (2014). *Speaking for patients and carers: Health consumer groups and the policy process*. New York: Macmillan.

Baggott, R., & Forster, R. (2008). Health consumer and patients' organizations in Europe: Towards a comparative analysis. *Health Expectations*, *11*(1), 85–94.

Barry, M. M., Domegan, C., Higgins, O., & Sixsmith, J. (2011). A literature review on health information seeking behaviour on the web: A health consumer and health professional perspective. *ECDC*. Retrieved from https://aran.library.nuigalway.ie/xmlui/bitstream/handle/10379/4588/Literature_review_on_health_information-seeking_behaviour_on_the_web.pdf?sequence=1

Bawden, D. (2001). Information overload. *Library & Information Briefings*, (92), 1–15.

Bawden, D., & Robinson, L. (2009). The dark side of information: Overload, anxiety and other paradoxes and pathologies. *Journal of Information Science*, *35*(2), 180–191.

Bennett, C., Graham, I. D., Kristjansson, E., Kearing, S. A., Clay, K. F., & O'Connor, A. M. (2010). Validation of a preparation for decision making scale. *Patient Education and Counseling*, *78*(1), 130–133. http://doi.org/10.1016/j.pec.2009.05.012.

Benzanson, B. J., & James, S. (2007). Culture-general and culture-specific approaches to counselling: Complementary stances. *International Journal for the Advancement of Counselling*, *29*, 159–171.

Blake, C. R., & Morey, M. R. (2000). Morningstar ratings and mutual fund performance. *Journal of Financial and Quantitative Analysis*, *35*(3), 451–483.

Bleakley, A. (2010). Blunting Occam's razor: Aligning medical education with studies of complexity. *Journal of Evaluation in Clinical Practice*, *16*, 849–855.

Blumer, H. (1969). *Symbolic interactionism: Perspective and method* (1st ed.). Berkeley, CA: University of California Press.

Bojuwoye, O. (2001). Crossing cultural boundaries in counseling. *International Journal for the Advancement of Counseling*, *23*, 31–50.

Brailsworth, S., Silverman, E., Rossiter, S., Bijak, J, Shaw, R., Viana, J., Noble, J., Efstathiou, S., & Vlachantoni, A. (2011). Complex systems modelling for supply and demand in health and social care. *Proceedings of the 2011 Winter Simulation Conference*. University of Southampton, Southampton.

Brunette, M. F., Gunn, W., Alvarez, H., Finn, P. C., Geiger, P., Ferron, J. C., & McHugo, G. J. (2015). A pre-post pilot study of a brief, web-based intervention to engage disadvantaged smokers into cessation treatment. *Addiction Science & Clinical Practice*, *10*(1), 1–8.

Cheng, F. K., & Tse, S. (2014). The use of Chinese Buddhist theories in counselling, psychotherapy, psychology, and mental health research: An integrative review. *International Journal for the Advancement of Counselling*, *36*, 229–242.

Coulter, A. (1998). Evidence based patient information: Is important, so there needs to be a national strategy to ensure it. *BMJ: British Medical Journal*, *317*(7153), 225.

Dalma, A., Karnaki, P., Zota, D., Veloudaki, A., Ellis-Montalban, P., Dotsikas, K., Christophi, C. A., Ioannidou, E., Patouris, E., Themistokleous, S., Batury, V., Linke, M., Berth, H., Sakowski, P., Darias-Curvo, S., & Linos, A. (2020). Physician-patient communication: A qualitative study of perceptions, barriers, and needs in four European member states. *Journal of Communication in Healthcare*, *13*(4), 301–313.

De Leo, G., LeRouge, C., Ceriani, C., & Niederman, F. (2006). Websites most frequently used by physician for gathering medical information. *AMIA Annual Symposium Proceedings* (Vol. 2006, p. 902). American Medical Informatics Association, Rockville, MD.

de Meyrick, J. (2003). The Delphi method and health research. *Health Education*, *103*(1), 7–16.

Dennis, A., & Martin, P. (2005). Symbolic interactionism and the concept of power. *British Journal of Sociology*, *56*(2), 191–213.

Department of Health. (2000). *NHS plan: A plan for investment, a plan for reform*. London: The Stationery Office.

Dev, R., Woods, N. F., Unger, J. A., Kinuthia, J., Matemo, D., Farid, S., Begnel, E. R., Kohler, P., & Drake, A. L. (2019). Acceptability, feasibility and utility of a mobile health family planning decision aid for postpartum women in Kenya. *Reproductive Health*, *16*(1), 1–11.

Doll, W. E. Jr, & Trueit, D. (2010). Complexity and the health care professions. *Journal of Evaluation in Clinical Practice*, *16*, 841–848.

Edmunds, A., & Morris, A. (2000). The problem of information overload in business organisations: A review of the literature. *International Journal of Information Management*, *20*(1), 17–28.

Eppler, M. J., & Mengis, J. (2004). The concept of information overload: A review of literature from organization science, accounting, marketing, MIS, and related disciplines. *The Information Society*, *20*(5), 325–344.

Eysenbach, G., & Jadad, A. R. (2001). Evidence-based patient choice and consumer health informatics in the Internet age. *Journal of Medical Internet Research*, *3*(2).

Flay, B. R., Biglan, A., Boruch, R. F., Castro, F. G., Gottfredson, D., Kellam, S., Mościcki, E., Schinke, S., Valentine, J. C., & Ji, P. (2005). Standards of evidence: Criteria for efficacy, effectiveness and dissemination. *Prevention Science*, *6*(3), 151–175.

Fowler, F. J., Levin, C. A., & Sepucha, K. R. (2011). Informing and involving patients to improve the quality of medical decisions. *Health Affairs*, *30*(4), 699–706.

Gallego, D., Woerndl, W., & Huecas, G. (2013). Evaluating the impact of proactivity in the user experience of a context-aware restaurant recommender for Android smartphones. *Journal of Systems Architecture*, *59*(9), 748–758.

Hall, A., & Walton, G. (2004). Information overload within the health care system: A literature review. *Health Information & Libraries Journal*, *21*(2), 102–108.

Higgins, J. P., Thompson, S. G., Deeks, J. J., & Altman, D. G. (2003). Measuring inconsistency in meta-analyses. *BMJ: British Medical Journal*, *327*(7414), 557.

Hopkin, G., Au, A., Collier, V. J., Yudkin, J. S., Basu, S., & Naci, H. (2019). Combining multiple treatment comparisons with personalized patient preferences: A randomized trial of an interactive platform for statin treatment selection. *Medical Decision Making*, *39*(3), 264–277.

Imai, K., Tingley, D., & Yamamoto, T. (2013). Experimental designs for identifying causal mechanisms. *Journal of the Royal Statistical Society: Series A (Statistics in Society)*, *176*(1), 5–51.

Ishikawa, H., Kawakami, N., Kessler, R. C., & World Mental Health Japan Survey Collaborators. (2016). Lifetime and 12-month prevalence, severity and unmet need for treatment of common mental disorders in Japan: Results from the final dataset of World Mental Health Japan Survey. *Epidemiology and Psychiatric Sciences*, *25*(3), 217–229.

Kirsch, D. (2000). A few thoughts on cognitive overload. *Intellectica*, *30*, 19–51.

Lamont, M. (2000). Meaning-making in cultural sociology: Broadening our agenda. *Contemporary Sociology*, *29*(4), 602–607.

Landeta, J. (2006). Current validity of the Delphi method in social sciences. *Technological Forecasting and Social Change*, *73*(5), 467–482.

Landy, R., Cameron, C., Au, A., Cameron, D., O'Brien, K., Robrigado, K., Baxter, L., Cockburn, L., O'Hearn, S., Oliver, B., & Nixon, S. A. (2016). Educational strategies to enhance reflexivity among clinicians and health professional students: A scoping study. *Forum: Qualitative Sozialforschung/Forum: Qualitative Social Research*, *17*(3), Article 14. Retrieved from www.qualitative-research.net/index.php/fqs/article/view/2573/4027

Linder, S. K., Swank, P. R., Vernon, S. W., Mullen, P. D., Morgan, R. O., & Volk, R. J. (2011). Validity of a low literacy version of the Decisional Conflict Scale. *Patient Education and Counseling*, *85*(3), 521–524. http://doi.org/10.1016/j.pec.2010.12.012

Litaker, D., Tomolo, A., Liberatore, V., Stange, K. C., & Aron, D. (2006). Using complexity theory to build interventions that improve health care delivery in primary care. *Journal of General Internal Medicine*, *21*, 30–34.

Liu, S. (2021). Between social spaces. *European Journal of Social Theory*, *24*(1), 123–139.

Loughran, K. (2016). Imbricated spaces: The high line, urban parks, and the cultural meaning of city and nature. *Sociological Theory*, *34*(4), 311–334.

Luo, A., He, H., Mohamed, S., & Rosenheck, R. (2018). Medical student attitudes towards people with mental illness in China: A qualitative study. *Culture, Medicine, and Psychiatry*, *42*(3), 535–551.

McMullan, M. (2006). Patients using the Internet to obtain health information: How this affects the patient–health professional relationship. *Patient Education and Counseling*, *63*(1–2), 24–28.

Mennin, S. (2010a). Complexity and health professions education. *Journal of Evaluation in Clinical Practice*, *16*, 835–837.

Mennin, S. (2010b). Self-organisation, integration and curriculum in the complex world of medical education. *Medical Education*, *44*, 20–30.

Morrison, K. (2005). Structuration theory, habitus, and complexity theory: Elective affinities or old wine in new bottles? *British Journal of Sociology of Education*, *26*(3), 311–326.

Moyo, F., Archibald, E., & Slyer, J. T. (2018). Effectiveness of decision aids for smoking cessation in adults: A quantitative systematic review. *JBI Evidence Synthesis*, *16*(9), 1791–1822.

Mullins, C. (2015, July). Responsive, mobile app, mobile first: Untangling the UX design web in practical experience. *Proceedings of the 33rd Annual International Conference on the Design of Communication* (pp. 1–6). Association for Computing Machinery, New York.

Munday, D. F., Johnson, S., & Griffiths, F. (2003). Complexity theory and palliative care. *Palliative Medicine*, *17*, 308–309.

Naci, H., Brugts, J. J., & Ades, T. (2013). Comparative tolerability and harms of individual statins : A study-level network meta-analysis of 246 955 participants from 135 randomized, controlled trials. *Circulation: Cardiovascular Quality and Outcomes*, *6*(4), 390–399. http://doi.org/10.1161/CIRCOUTCOMES.111.000071

Naci, H., Brugts, J. J., Fleurence, R., Tsoi, B., Toor, H., & Ades, A. E. (2013). Comparative benefits of statins in the primary and secondary prevention of major coronary events and all-cause mortality: A network meta-analysis of placebo-controlled and active-comparator trials. *European Journal of Preventive Cardiology*, *20*(4), 641–657. http://doi.org/10.1177/2047487313480435

Naci, H., & Ioannidis, J. P. (2015). Evaluation of wellness determinants and interventions by citizen scientists. *JAMA*, *314*(2), 121–122.

Nagar, S. (2022). The struggle of mental health care delivery in South Korea and Singapore. *Harvard International Review*. Retrieved from https://hir.harvard.edu/the-struggle-of-mental-health-care-delivery-in-south-korea-and-singapore/

Nilsen, E. S., Myrhaug, H. T., Johansen, M., Oliver, S., & Oxman, A. D. (2006). Methods of consumer involvement in developing healthcare policy and research, clinical practice guidelines and patient information material. *Cochrane Database of Systematic Reviews*, *3*(3).

Nimmon, L., & Stenfors-Hayes, T. (2016). The "handling" of power in the physician-patient encounter: Perceptions from experienced physicians. *BMC Medical Education*, *16*(1), 114.

O'Connor, A. M. (1995). *User manual – decision self-efficacy scale*. Ottawa: The Ottawa Hospital.

O'Connor, A. M., Legare, F., Lewis, K., Barry, M., Bennett, C. L., Eden, K. B., Holmes-Rovner, M., Llewellyn-Thomas, H., Lyddiatt, A., Thomson, R., & Trevena, L. (2017). Decision aids for people facing health treatment or screening decisions. *Cochrane Database of Systematic Reviews, (4)*. Retrieved from www.cochranelibrary.com/cdsr/doi/10.1002/14651858.CD001431.pub5/full

O'Connor, A. M., Rostom, A., Fiset, V., Tetroe, J., Entwistle, V., Llewellyn-Thomas, H., Holmes-Rovner, M., Barry, M., & Jones, J. (1999). Decision aids for patients facing health treatment or screening decisions: Systematic review. *BMJ*, *319*(7212), 731–734.

Oliver, K. A., de Vocht, F., Money, A., & Everett, M. (2017). Identifying public health policymakers' sources of information: Comparing survey and network analyses. *European Journal of Public Health*, *27*(Suppl. 2), 118–123.

Or, C. K., & Karsh, B. T. (2009). A systematic review of patient acceptance of consumer health information technology. *Journal of the American Medical Informatics Association*, *16*(4), 550–560.

Paley, J. (2010). The appropriation of complexity theory in health care. *Journal of Health Services Research & Policy*, *15*(1), 59–61.

Pedersen, P. B. (1997). The cultural context of the American Counseling Association code of ethics. *Journal of Counseling & Development*, *76*(1), 23–28.

Que, J., Lu, L., & Shi, L. (2019). Development and challenges of mental health in China. *General Psychiatry*, *32*(1), e100053.

Rawson, M. (2010). *Eden on the Charles: The making of Boston*. Cambridge, MA: Harvard University Press.

Sanson-Fisher, R. W., Bonevski, B., Green, L. W., & D'Este, C. (2007). Limitations of the randomized controlled trial in evaluating population-based health interventions. *American Journal of Preventive Medicine*, *33*(2), 155–161.

Schwartz, B., Ward, A., Monterosso, J., Lyubomirsky, S., White, K., & Lehman, D. (2002). Maximizing versus satisficing: Happiness is a matter of choice. *Journal of Personality and Social Psychology*, *83*(5), 1178.

Simmel, G. (1997). Money and commodity culture. In D. Frisby & M. Featherstone (Eds.), *Simmel on culture* (Ch.8). London: SAGE. (Original work published 1900)

Singal, A. G., Higgins, P. D., & Waljee, A. K. (2014). A primer on effectiveness and efficacy trials. *Clinical and Translational Gastroenterology*, *5*(1), e45.

Sparling, E. I., & Sen, S. (2011, October). Rating: How difficult is it? *Proceedings of the Fifth ACM Conference on Recommender Systems* (pp. 149–156). Association for Computing Machinery, New York.

Speier, C., Valacich, J. S., & Vessey, I. (1999). The influence of task interruption on individual decision making: An information overload perspective. *Decision Sciences*, *30*(2), 337–360.

Stacey, D., Légaré, F., & Lewis, K. B. (2017). Patient decision aids to engage adults in treatment or screening decisions. *JAMA*, *318*(7), 657–658.

Stefanovics, E. A., Rosenheck, R. A., He, H., Ofori-Atta, A., Cavalcanti, M., & Chiles, C. (2016). Medical student beliefs and attitudes toward mental illness across five nations. *Journal of Nervous and Mental Disease*, *204*(12), 909–915.

Stewart, M. A. (1995). Effective physician-patient communication and health outcomes: A review. *CMAJ: Canadian Medical Association Journal*, *152*(9), 1423.

Tatman, A. (2004). Hmong history, culture and acculturation: Implications for counseling the Hmong. *Journal of Multicultural Counseling and Development*, *32*, 222–234.

Tso, P., Culyer, A. J., Brouwers, M., & Dobrow, M. J. (2011). Developing a decision aid to guide public sector health policy decisions: A study protocol. *Implementation Science*, *6*(1), 1–5.

Wampold, B. E. (2001). *The great psychotherapy debate: Models, methods and findings*. Mahwah, NJ: Erlbaum.

Willemsen, M. C., Wiebing, M., Van Emst, M. A., & Zeeman, G. (2006). Helping smokers to decide on the use of efficacious smoking cessation methods: A randomized controlled trial of a decision aid. *Addiction, 101*(3), 441–449.

World Health Organization. (2008). *The global burden of disease*. Geneva: Author.

World Health Organization. (2019). *The WHO special initiative for mental health (2019–2023): Universal health coverage for mental health*. Geneva: Author. Retrieved from https://apps.who.int/iris/bitstream/handle/10665/310981/WHO-MSD-19.1-eng.pdf?sequence=1&isAllowed=y

Zhou, F., Ji, Y., & Jiao, R. J. (2014). Prospect-theoretic modeling of customer affective-cognitive decisions under uncertainty for user experience design. *IEEE Transactions on Human-Machine Systems, 44*(4), 468–483.

Zhu, Y., Zhang, H., Yang, G., Hu, X., Liu, Z., Guo, N., He, H., Sun, B., & Rosenheck, R. (2018). Attitudes towards mental illness among medical students in China: Impact of medical education on stigma. *Asia-Pacific Psychiatry, 10*(2), e12294.

6 Cultural Beliefs and Social Media

The Rise and Study of Social Media

Over the past decade since the conception of social media, their use has proliferated across the globe. People have been logging in, posting content, building relationships with other people, and populating the online sphere of social media in modern apps, such as Instagram, Facebook, WeChat, Kakao, LINE, and Weibo. The sheer growth in social media users in the region has been unprecedented.

Figure 6.1 shows the extent of this proliferation in absolute terms with the number of social media users in millions in East Asia. The region witnessed significant annual increases in the number of users in just the past five years. From 2017 to 2021, China grew from 684 million users to about 1 billion users, Japan grew from 63.68 million users to 96.95 million users, and South Korea grew from 40.24 million users to 45.58 million users.

China and Japan both averaged double-digit gains annually, about 10% and 11%, respectively, in the growth of the number of users over the past five years. Though the number of users in South Korea grew noticeably slower, averaging around 3% per year, all countries were home to a large number of users in relative terms.

Figure 6.2 shows the number of social media users as a proportion of the general population in each of the three countries. As we can see, the proportion of users is highest in South Korea, growing from 78.35% to 87.96% of the population, followed by Japan, which grew from 50.22% to 77.31%, and China, which also skyrocketed from 49.37% to 70.92%. In just five years' time, about three-quarters or more of the general population in East Asia have come online to use social media.

The study of social media has stimulated important lines of inquiry on these user behaviors, with particular attention to online and offline interpersonal interactions (Tian, 2017), how users build their identities online (Robinson, 2007), and the way users present themselves (boyd, 2006; boyd & Heer, 2006), calling into account symbolic interactionist accounts of presentation and self-censorship (Marwick & boyd, 2010).

DOI:10.4324/9781003308720-6

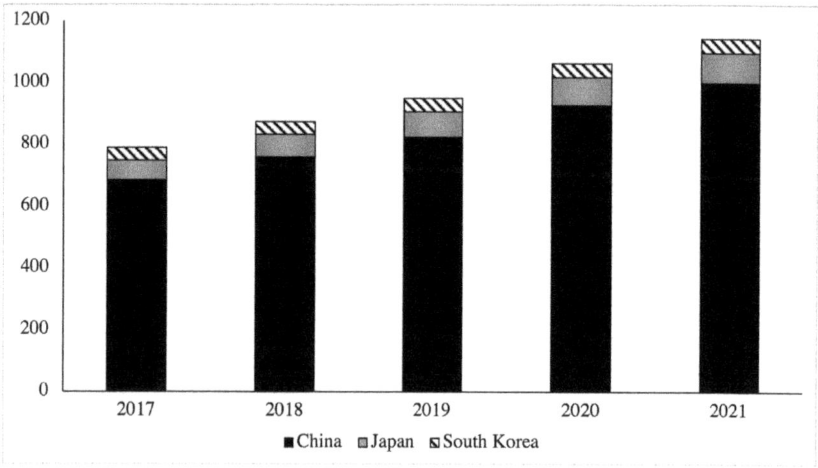

Figure 6.1 Number of social media users (millions) by country in China, Japan, and South Korea.

Sources: Jobst (2021), Lai (2021), Statista Research Department (2021)

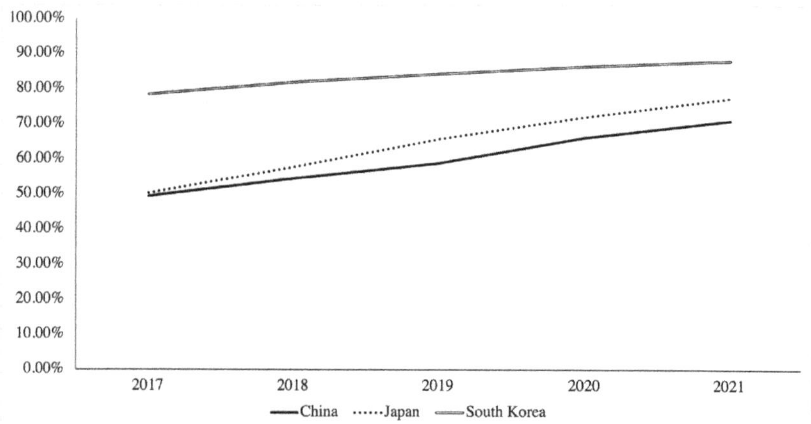

Figure 6.2 Number of social media users as a proportion of the general population in China, Japan, and South Korea.

Sources: Jobst (2021), Lai (2021), Statista Research Department (2021)

Much of this research has evidently focused on the way social media use shapes instrumental action in interacting with others and producing content as members of a network.

This chapter examines how social media similarly affects the way we feel. That is, the same social mechanisms by which social media affects the way we act lend well to governing our emotions (see Ben-Ze'ev, 2004; Gonzalez-Polledo & Tarr, 2016; Lieberman & Goldstein, 2006).

Internet communications create and modulate collective emotional states, through pathways of social influence similar to contagion in social networks (Onnela & Reed-Tsochas, 2010; Szell et al., 2010). Within this scope, some online communities have been found to be sustained by emotional expressiveness itself (Chmiel et al., 2011a, 2011b). Emotions are typically expressed using combinations of non-linguistic mechanisms, such as smiling, vocal intonation, and facial expressions. However, evidence shows that textual communication can proffer modes of expression no less rich, and which are augmented by expressive textual methods embedded in social media functions, such as emoticons and slang (Gamon et al., 2005).

This chapter takes this as a starting point to examine how emotions affect user behaviors and how emotions are fundamentally expressed within social media platforms. This chapter focuses on the kinds of emotional labor that people perform. Emotional labor is classically defined as the management of emotions in the context of one's social roles, often including work roles (Grandey, 2000), which finds strong convergences with the various social roles folded into one identity among users online (Ritzer & Jurgenson, 2010). Users, for instance, are producers of content; at the same time they are consumers, as well as friends with fellow producers and consumers.

This chapter reflects on in-depth interviews with Hong Kong and mainland Chinese university students to explore how emotions are conveyed and perceived in social media use, and in doing so, elaborate on the normative, rational strategies with which emotional labor is conducted in the context of users' overlapping social roles.

In so doing, this chapter inductively characterizes three types of strategies. (1) strategies employed to manage *emotional reactions*, centering on norms about likable and dislikable emotions. Here, I draw upon the concept of critical distance from sociology of culture to interpret strategies used to circumvent emotional exhaustion from dislikable emotions and content overload. (2) Strategies to manage *emotional conveyances*, particularly as users attempt to navigate norms of emotional perception, such as manipulating the temporality of posts to express dislikable emotions without incurring backlash. I extrapolate from the concept of imagined audience to formulate imagined competition and imagined content. (3) The combination of these sets of strategic behaviors to facilitate the creation of a Simmelian digital blasé anchored in a layered *emotional detachment* into which all users are inevitably pulled.

The Labor of Viewing Content: Managing Critical Distance and Emotional Reaction

Emotions have been afforded an incredibly diverse set of definitions. This chapter will build upon emotions defined as (a) "appraisals of a situational stimulus," and (b) "the display of expressive gestures" (Thoits, 1989, p. 318), with particular focus on feelings, the experience of an emotional state, particularly positive and negative feelings, such as happiness, sadness, and fear; moods, chronic states of feeling that may or may not be embedded in a social context; and sentiments, which are "socially constructed pattern[s] of sensations, expressive gestures, and cultural meanings organized around a relationship to a social object, usually another person . . . or group such as a family" (Gordon, 1981, pp. 566–567). These forms of emotions are managed in terms of content viewed (emotional reaction) and content produced (emotional conveyance), strategies within which work toward creating a digital blasé, whose emotional detachment perforates the atmosphere of social media.

Users regularly felt inundated with an overload of content, coming to expect it every time they logged in and viewed social media. Even among those who used social media as often as six to eight hours a day felt unable to keep up and properly process all the material they viewed. As Yang Min, a 20-year-old female student, notes,

> I think there are too many news and comments on the social media. I think if you want to pay attention to every comment, it's too [tiring]. . . . I would feel more emotionally exhausted if I had to care about so much stuff. So I don't care about it.

This inundation could be sourced to two practices universal among social media users. First, users made use of the freedom to express and seek out content on social media by following a range of personal interests and public figures, including beauty, cosmetics, fashion, lifestyle, food, political and tabloid news, travel, and celebrities. Second, users reported treating social media as "modern-day phonebooks" with which to keep in contact with others they meet and wish to keep in touch with, anticipating an inflation in one's friends lists and following counts and, by extension, in the amount of content one saw online.

Indeed, the task of investing oneself in the content one saw, enough to reflect upon and stimulate an emotional reaction, constituted an impossible task by virtue of the sheer volume of posts that was ever-growing and ever-changing. Yet, the shape of this indifference was not molded by the refusal of emotional investment/reaction alone. A second, more powerful influence arose from others, whose co-present identities were inextricably tied to the content that one saw, coming to reshape its subjectivity in ways that distanced content producer from content viewer. Presented with content overload, users felt a need to be more selective about the material they allowed themselves to feel invested in, making selective cuts to content. The criteria that guided these "cuts" figured around content deemed irrelevant to their social lives, such as (1) posts that were made by contacts, rather than friends and, related, (2) those that lacked utility.

Putting (1) in network terms, users restricted their attention to content generated by their stronger ties, filtering out content made by weaker ones. In Yang Min's own words, this was "because I think it's another's life and far from me. And it's not my business, so it won't affect me very much." These sentiments were echoed by Lee, a 20-one-year-old female, who reported an overarching sense of apathy that was difficult to break:

Lee: I feel more neutral. I guess consistently more numb on Instagram. Even Facebook is boring too, because what I find really interesting . . . maybe there [are only a few] posts that I really think that are interesting.
Interviewer: You said you used Facebook to read news though. What about that?
Lee: I think it's just informative, but not interesting.

Yet, the apathy was not impenetrable. Or rather, *when* a user's apathy could *not* be broken was made possible by its factoring into the same calculations for when apathy *could* be broken, as with friends. The powerful of the distinction between friends (stronger ties) and contacts who users did not know very well (weaker ties), embodying a difference between allowed and forbidden subjective emotional investment, was captured by Vivian, another 21-year-old female:

> It's only my friends [that makes me care]. If after I see my friend's pages, I see the others one sadness or happiness, I think it is not my business. I can use another angle to recognize or know more about that [person], but for me, *no matter how the person* is happy or sad, it's not my business. I can't do anything about that person or I *won't want* to do anything for that person. So I [am] numb.

Thus, (2) no matter how grave the material presented, so long as it was not relevant to the user through practical utility or association with their stronger ties, it was insufficient to overcome apathy and invoke emotional investment. That is, something could be seen as useful if it was related to one's friends – the utility in such an arrangement lies in the preservation of a social relationship. Moreover, the nature of this apathy was rooted in a reflexive practice of formulating a critical distance toward others.

From the sociology of culture, critical distance is a mode of cultural evaluation and epistemic virtue characterized by a critical autonomy and a balance between distance and engagement (Chong, 2013). It is typically leveraged to transform tastes into reasoned and legitimate representations of a product. Applied to social media, critical distance is similarly employed among users toward posts, to present emotional values and tastes in rational terms. Within this scope, the emotional content of an "irrelevant" post is alienated and denied by its subsumption into objectivized calculations built upon critical autonomy and a reflexive reading of content, measured against one's position (Jerolmack & Khan, 2014; Landy et al., 2016). Such values were rooted in self-interests, for instance, enacted by alienating content to prevent emotional investment and, by extension, disappointment. Critical distance, thus, was sometimes an act of self-protection. As Chen, an 18-year-old male, shows, emotional apathy was sometimes *triggered by* emotional investment in friends' content as a result of jealousy and a defensive reaction to it:

> I feel numb [when using social media usually]. I get annoyed if there are too many photos of friends traveling, and I can't travel, and they're posting so many photos online [*laughs*], and I get annoyed. It's called *saiban* ["washing over everything you see in a page"] and I can't see other stuff and it makes me feel so annoyed. I really don't feel anything.

Thus, although Chen was privy to a general emotional apathy, emotional investment actually predicted apathy during moments where the practices embedded in content clashed with his values about relative deprivation: liking and being unable to travel, yet forced to witness others doing what he cannot do. Apathy was a self-defense mechanism for thwarting the annoyance or turmoil brought on by such value clashes. Furthermore, Chen's values were bound up in emotional perception, resonating with larger attempts to regulate one's emotional reactions to material by censoring and filtering content visible in the first place.

Users were accustomed to possessing and exercising control over the content presented to them through public pages for personal interests, such as news and media, lifestyle and entertainment, among others. Whenever clashes of values erupted within this arrangement, users would simply unfollow the pages, essentially severing connections between them. For friends and contacts, however, users were unable to exercise such a practice, even when faced with such clashes; doing so was taken to mean a severance of a tie – a drastic measure that threatened to destroy the dyadic relationship. As such, value clashes were accommodated for by leveraging emotional apathy, innately tied to the practice of regulating one's emotions in terms of the content one emotionally responds to. For instance, Wing, a 20-year-old female, described her aversion to a particular type of content:

Wing: I avoid selfies. I don't post selfies.
Interviewer: Why is that?
Wing: Well, I think it's too confident.
Interviewer: Too confident. Okay, so what do you think when other people post selfies?
Wing: Depends if the person is beautiful and handsome, or not. If not, then I think it's too confident. [*laughs*]
Interviewer: Okay. You think, "they shouldn't be on Instagram."
Wing: Yeah. [*laughs*] Instagram police . . .

But as much as Wing "policed" selfie posts whenever she came across them, she did not make known her feelings. Rather, she chose to ignore them, as well as the users responsible for posting them, ultimately relying on emotional apathy and critical distance to manage potential emotional discomfort and prevent a falling out.

Ranee, a 19-year-old female, reported a similar sentiment: "I think [sad things] are annoying. . . . I have a friend who posts sad things all the time, every day, and I think it's annoying." Ranee later clarified in the dialogue that "annoying" referred to a much more personal level of discomfort, citing mental health as a concern. But even as she felt this way, as the value clash between producer and viewer figured around health rather than taste, Ranee did as Wing, Chen, and others (whose value clashes *were* simply differences in taste) did: prioritize the maintenance of the relationship, whose value derived from its roots in the "real world," above personal discomfort in the "online world." In this way, emotional investment in friends' content can precede apathy and critical distance, not as a mode of condescension but as a way of protecting oneself and the relationship.

The Labor of Posting Content: Managing Temporality and Emotional Conveyance

In addition to managing what one viewed, users also managed what they themselves posted. Apart from sensitive topics for fear of backlash, such as politics or religion (Marwick & boyd, 2010), emotions themselves became subjects of self-censorship. Moreover, just as emotional reactions were managed through subjective selection and reinterpretation of content, *conveyances* of emotion were also intensely managed. Emotional apathy is a set of strategic, calculated reactions to value clashes during emotional investment. In particular, Ranee's case shows how emotions themselves can be implicated in these clashes. My dialogue with Wing reveals how these strategies and perceptions surface in the reverse position and, intriguingly, how specific features of Instagram reshape them:

Interviewer: Some people avoid posting about negative feelings or negative experiences. . . . [D]o you feel that as well?

Wing: Sometimes I post negative things . . . because I want my friends know that I'm feeling sad now. And maybe they can help me and they can give me some comfort.

Interviewer: How would you post that?

Wing: I would post that on my Instagram story. Something that *disappears*.

The Instagram story is a function that allows users to post pictures or videos on one's profile, but which is only visible to one's followers and for 24 hours before it automatically deletes itself. Features of social media enabled users to manage a new element: temporality. Wing emphasized how the story provided a tool that allowed her to capture her feelings, and whose transience enabled her to express them in a socially acceptable way while reaching out for social support from her network. Reflecting on the difference between the Instagram story and an actual post, Wing also elaborates on the distinct interpretations imbued to permanent and transient forms of content:

Interviewer: Would you ever post something sad on your actual profile then?
Wing: Actual profile, no.
Interviewer: Why is that?
Wing: I think I want my profile to be happier . . . I want to maintain a happy image.
Interviewer: Why?
Wing: I think maybe I want my life to be happy. Yes. I think if post it on the story, then it would be gone soon. And maybe if I post it, my sadness will be gone so soon too.
Interviewer: Does the fact that other people are watching your profile make a difference?
Wing: Yes. I don't post something unhappy because I think it will *last*. And people will see that and they think I am un unhappy person. I don't want people to think I am unhappy. I think I want to have an image that I am happy in my every day. Something like that.
Interviewer: Why do you want that image though?
Wing: It is to be liked. Maybe if I'm more positive, people will like me more.

Reinforcing what Ranee also pointed out as the need to maintain a happy image, Wing felt compelled to self-censor negative parts of her life from public expression on her profile through posts, driven by fear of incurring backlash or social disapproval. This resonates with a dramaturgical management of one's sense of self (Vaccaro et al., 2011), wherein emotional work is shaped by needs and norms of social appearance. Lee, a 21-year-old female, further illuminated the contours of the influence and consequences emotional content held within the online community.

Interviewer: And why is it that you feel you need to maintain a happy image?
Lee: I think a post has an influence on other people. If my posts are very pessimistic, they will make the one who sees them unhappy, or also think negatively.

Interviewer: What makes you care about that?
Lee: Because my personality is [like] this. Because I, hmm, from my very young age, I already have this personality, to care more other feelings rather than my own feelings.

Lee's calculated decision to self-censor her pessimistic posts resulted from a grounded interpretation of emotional discharge as socially contagious. This adds insight to recent quantitative studies and field experiments of online social contagion, which demonstrate that social contagion only operates through dissemination of information, with little capacity to motivate action, such as fundraising (Lacetera et al., 2016). Yet, respondents in this study highlight a third, neglected dimension through which social contagion operates: the contagion of emotions (feelings).

Gamson, a 24-year-old male, rehashes a similar sentiment about how happiness is no less contagious than pessimism: "when I see they are very interesting, I feel sad. And maybe [if posts and other users are happy and] I also read this, I think at that time I will feel happy." Viewing emotional content invoked similar feelings in viewers, an effect mediated by the general sentiment of social approval toward happiness and disapproval toward pessimism, as well as the perceived purpose of social media as a space of relaxation by users.

Simultaneously, Wing's calculated decision to express her feelings through a story, rather than a post, throws into sharp relief the perceived risks of permanence with which things collect and linger in perpetuity for judgment by oneself and others. Choosing a permanent mode of expression for negative feelings risked resurrecting the very same feelings captured in the particular post when one looked back at it in the future; at the same time it risked transforming the user into a person who was disapproved of and evoked critical distance from others who, like Ranee, found negative things annoying and disturbing.

Interestingly, even Ranee herself made use of the story to express her unhappy feelings, which she described:

> [S]ometimes I like writing my own feelings or jotting down my feelings when I feel sad. But I don't want everybody to know that, and I need some channel to express it – so that's the twenty-four-hour story.

Reconciling her need to express or vent her feelings with her recognition of how too much negative expression can be annoying, Ranee resorted to using the story – something that was restricted in its reach and temporary in its form. Thus, the management of feelings and their expression needed to account for popularized, disapproving sentiments about negativity itself. More importantly, this management encompassed sets of strategies to manipulate content that users viewed, as well as that which they produced, both of which often overlapped and mediated one another.

The Labor of Sustaining Emotion: Managing Emotional Indifference and the Digital Blasé

Underpinning the management of emotional reaction and conveyance was a general mood of indifference that users entered into social media with, which, combined with a reported overload of content, lays the foundation for a digital blasé. According to Simmel (1903/1976), the blasé consists of an attitude of general indifference, which arises as a psychological reaction to mass stimulation emotionally generated through media and the co-presence of others:

> The psychological foundation, upon which the metropolitan individuality is erected, is the intensification of emotional life due to the swift and continuous shift of external and internal stimuli. . . . Lasting *impressions*, the slightness in their differences, the habituated regularity of their course and contrasts between them, consume, so to speak, less mental energy than the rapid telescoping of changing images, pronounced differences within what is grasped at a single glance, and the unexpectedness of violent stimuli . . . the metropolis creates these psychological conditions – with every crossing of the street, with the tempo and multiplicity of economic, occupational and social life.
>
> (Simmel, 1903/1976, pp. 409–410, italics added)

Social media studies corroborate the investment of emotions in internet exchanges (Chmiel et al., 2011a, 2011b) but built upon the presupposition of social media as visualizations of our physical networks. But as users point out, online social life consists of more than interactions with our friends and acquaintances; or rather, our online networks are comprised also by our participation in or observation of public pages that express personal interests.

As Simmel describes, the theoretical purchase of the blasé is represented by continual exposure to stimulating content that *overstimulates* us to the effect of generating widespread emotional detachment. As such, it means we feel less attached, as well as the need to actively avoid engagement altogether, organized around a need to censor interaction or expressions, further reflected among users. Thus, the overload of online content and the consequences it holds for interactions on social media crystallize a digital blasé in three ways, in which norms of emotional reaction and conveyance are bound up: emotional detachment, the perceived need to detach, and a sense of watchedness.

Users described the atmosphere of social media in terms of mood and inclination toward a particular feeling, which was further distinguished between Facebook and Instagram. According to Esther, a 21-year-old female:

Esther: [Facebook and Instagram are] very different.
Interviewer: Can you tell me more?
Esther: On Instagram, the atmosphere is good, because . . . the people I follow and the people who follow me are my friends. So I think the comments are very positive. Like you post a travelling photo and my friends will say "oh it's beautiful," something like that. But I think on Facebook, there are very negative comments, like a political issue . . . there are some people [who] . . . just want to complain, complain, and complain.

Instagram's atmosphere or mood was more consistent with Esther's expectations of social media as a tool for leisure. Her depiction of these expectations also uncovered a specific form of emotional detachment from certain types of content (political commentary and opinions), which also resonated with a general aversion to politics and the need to ignore such content. Elaborating on a more general form of this detachment, or a mood that hung around specific social media, Cheung, a 19-year-old female, describes:

Cheung: I think that people usually talk about serious stuff on Facebook, rather than Instagram. On Instagram . . . everything's relaxing – hanging out with friends, events where you're really enjoy[ing] the event, or if people post a lot of photos about travel.
Interviewer: So you see a lot of happy stuff . . . do your emotions fluctuate?
Cheung: I would say I'm more numb . . . When I see something happy, I feel happy. But when I see something unhappy, I will try to think what I can do.
Interviewer: But you wouldn't feel very unhappy.
Cheung: I think you have to face problems if you keep avoiding it you can't solve it.

Like Esther, Cheung felt that Facebook embodied an atmosphere that evoked a more serious mood,[1] which went against her desire to use social media for leisure, better captured by Instagram. Furthermore, she also felt that Facebook's stern gravity consisted of the tendency to complain, wherein pessimism better resembled inaction than expression. But in her dialogue, numbness gained credence as a default state into which users entered upon logging into social media – and *to which* users returned.

The recursive transition back to numbness from feeling was facilitated directly and *indirectly* by an overload of content. On the one hand, users felt there was "too much to care about," as Yang Min noted, emphasizing "emotional exhaustion." In other cases, excessive content did not dull the tendency to feel among users but instead overstimulated them to the effect of shortening the lifespan of these emotions. For Julie, a 21-year-old female, feelings were easily "contracted" per social contagion, but easily purged:

Julie: I think I have more mood swings on Facebook. . . . [S] ometimes when I saw some very traumatic news, like the accident, something like that, I just feel sad.

Interviewer: What changes do you experience in your feelings?

Julie: Hmm?

Interviewer: Do your feelings go up, down, up, down?

Julie: [I think I'm] sad for a time and then I scroll, and when I see something happy, then I'm happier. . . . [My feelings] rarely last too long, unless I really see something related to me. Like my high school teacher passed away a few years ago. Then I felt I was sad for a longer time, but I don't think it's related to the posts. Because I can gain such information from other sources as well.

Interviewer: Okay. So it was more personal to you and it came from a real place for you, right?

Julie: Yeah. And you know, there are quite a lot of accidents happening every day. And you can't feel sad every time you see those posts. Maybe you will just feel, like you feel that they [deserve pity]. It won't affect my mood too much.

Content from posts rarely evoked emotional reactions among users per critical distance, which, as Julie indicates, stems from a state of emotional detachment. Furthermore, symptoms of the direct and indirect effects of content overload on blasé were visible, with "quite a lot of accidents happening every day" that drained users' capacity to feel, as well as the brevity with which emotions that they *did* feel lasted; posts, after all, were fated to replacement by the next in a perpetual tide of endless content ready to spring an exhausting array of feelings upon emotionally unprepared users. And as Gamson indicates:

> Like many people, I want to know more about what [my friends] are doing, about what their life is like. So I want to read their posts, [even though] I don't make posts. I feel I am *not* very happy. I am reading their posts and must feel very bored. Only when I'm very bored will I read this.

Thus, reversion to blasé was imminent and inevitable, coming to precede and succeed emotional interest in others. From Yang Min, we can infer how emotional detachment was a strategy to accommodate for content overload and prevent in advance the emotional exhaustion it would incur:

> I see a lot of happy things and unhappy things on social media right. My emotions are not up down up down, but . . . I will say numb. Because [there are] so many things. And they just . . . keep on repeating, and so I hate it. Because I've seen everything already.

Even though substantive forms and topics of posts tended to vary, to the extent that they produced an overload of content, Yang Min focused on the emotional content of posts to illustrate a more nuanced dimension of emotional exhaustion: how in spite of substantive differences in posts, the emotional reaction and wear they imposed were the same. Thus, the *repetition* of emotional reaction was conducive to emotional exhaustion, prompting the need to detach before the content is even seen. Drawing inspiration from the concept of imagined competitors or imagined audience (Litt, 2012) – mental conceptualizations of who we are interacting with, influencing our speech and actions – users generated a sense of *imagined content* defined by excess content, overstimulation, and emotional exhaustion, to which they anticipatorily reacted by generating emotional detachment before and during their social media use. Parallels can be drawn with findings from the study of risk emotions that empower this assertion: feelings of fear and anxiety arise from future-oriented projection of harm, be it physical or social, which spur attempts to preemptively manage their causes (Cottingham & Fisher, 2016).

Within a digital blasé, the co-presence of others, forming imagined audience and competitors, impressed a sense of watchedness upon social media users, which discouraged both emotional reaction and conveyance. Kwong, a 21-year-old female, noted how she felt uncomfortable to post "because everyone can see it. Because I added many friends that I basically don't know, just because they are mutual friends of one of my friends, so I add them." As a result, she felt she was always under surveillance:

Kwong: I feel I am being watched by people.
Interviewer: And why do you feel uncomfortable with people being able to see your stuff?
Kwong: I think it depends on what kind of stuff. Yeah, because . . . if my post directly refers to someone that I don't want him to see, then I will be very worried for him to see it.

It emerges that imagined audience, anchored in the co-presence of others, operated as a mechanism through which emotional detachment is established. Kwong was concerned about the visibility of her emotional expressions to imagined members of her own network, hearkening to the use of self-censorship. The boundaries of this imagined audience are far more expansive than personal networks, as Esther shows, coming to encompass the possibility of invisible strangers drifting in from uncharted seas of social media:

> If a lot of people followed me . . . a lot of people started watching me. I might start posting less. Maybe. Depends on what kinds of people follow me. If they are friends, then I don't mind. If they are strangers, I will post less photos.

The social construction of imagined audiences empowers the structure of the blasé. Where the concept of imagined audience holds that imagining characteristics of our audience shapes how we present ourselves, the blasé contextualizes this process with an atmosphere of emotional detachment, leveraging it to make sense of how social media users in Hong Kong have generally chosen to censor themselves. Furthermore, the pervasive sense of being watched was counterbalanced with how watching was the most reported activity among users themselves in their use of social media: passively scrolling and observing content, rather than producing it.

That is, users consistently reported feeling uncomfortable with posting, and even more so with leaving comments on public content, citing uncertainty about stranger reactions and fear of inciting arguments. Like influential outsiders who are silent observers or audience members in other digital contexts of interaction (Tian & Menchik, 2016), the silent, observing imagined audience in the digital blasé on social media wield tremendous influence over users, but which derives from the specter of their anonymous, implied presence, more than their actual interaction.

Indeed, it is the imagined backlash, which is ever-present, more than the actual backlash, which is rare, that shores suffering and urges the numbing of emotional expression and reaction. Thus, recasting the repertoire of posts made on online social media as a digital blasé, it emerges that the more users watch others online, the more users feel they themselves are being watched. As a result, they feel discouraged from investing themselves emotionally, and so work to reduce their engagement and participation online.

Social Media as a Turning Point

As Chapter 3 alluded, social media can facilitate the diffusion of information and ties with superior speed than in-person networks. The idea of watchedness discussed in this chapter also resonates with the embeddedness that Chapter 3 described as keeping East Asians beholden to cultural beliefs, for fear of being caught reneging on established norms and bringing dishonor to themselves or their families. Chapter 5 also touched upon the ways that social media can facilitate misinformation simply because there are fewer checks on the information being passed through them.

This chapter offers a counterpoint to these findings. It shows that, for all the ways that social media can entrench rather than resist cultural stigmatization against mental health, it also has the potential to socialize users into tapping into emotions rather than banishing them outright.

Negative emotions are shunned upon, while positive emotions are praised as the norm. At the same time, users suppress the negative content of their own emotional expressions or manipulate the temporality or lifespan of their content to successfully express negative emotions while navigating repressive norms about negativity. These, in turn, are anticipatory actions to help circumvent the emotional exhaustion believed to arise from imagined content. Furthermore, a digital blasé arises from these structured sets of behaviors that consists the general atmosphere of social media, sustained by three characteristics: emotional detachment, the perceived need for detachment, and a pervasive sense of watchedness. Users enter upon social media with a state of emotional detachment. Even if emotions are felt and emotional preparedness fails, they do not last long: users are not pulled from the blasé for long before they are inevitably returned to it, that is, to the numbness with which they began their use of social media.

This is significant in East Asian cultures that suppress emotions, as Chapter 2 described. Social media is imparting a newfound emotionality unto users, evinced by how different social medias are leveraged to manage and express emotions. The social mechanisms underpinning instrumental action and emotional labor are shared; that is, although much social media research exists to explicate the social norms governing interactions online, the emotional implications of posts often take precedence above their substance in determining how users post, comment, think, and feel.

Considering the sheer number of people flocking to social media in their everyday lives, we may be witnessing a gradual shift in the way cultural beliefs toward mental health, potentially for good, as discussed in this chapter, as much as for bad, as covered in the previous chapters. More broadly, this chapter also shows that emotions – or the lack thereof – not only present artifacts for inquiry in themselves but offer a powerful lens through which to visualize and make sense of habits and modes of thinking otherwise invisible in online networks formed on social media.

Note

1 Many other users also corroborated this sentiment.

References

Ben-Ze'ev, A. (2004). *Love online: Emotions on the Internet*. Cambridge: Cambridge University Press.

boyd, d. (2006). Friends, friendsters, and myspace top 8: Writing community into being on social network sites. *First Monday*, *11*(2). Retrieved from http://firstmonday.org/chapter/view/1418/1336

boyd, d., & Heer, J. (2006). Profiles as conversation: Networked identity performance on friendster. *Proceedings of the 39th Hawaii International Conference on System Sciences* (pp. 1–10). Institute of Electrical and Electronics Engineers Computer Society, Washington, DC.

Chmiel, A., Sienkiewicz, J., Thelwall, M., Paltoglou, G., Buckley, K., Kappas, A., & Hołyst, J. A. (2011b). Collective emotions online and their influence on community life. *PLoS One*, *6*(7), e22207.

Chmiel, A., Sobkowicz, P., Sienkiewicz, J., Paltoglou, G., Buckley, K., Thelwal, M., & Holyst, J. A. (2011a). Negative emotions boost user activity at BBC forum. *Physica A*, *390*, 2936–2944.

Chong, P. (2013). Legitimate judgment in art, the scientific world reversed? Maintaining critical distance in evaluation. *Social Studies of Science*, *43*(2), 265–281.

Cottingham, M. D., & Fisher, J. A. (2016). Risk and emotion among healthy volunteers in clinical trials. *Social Psychology Quarterly*, *79*(3), 222–242.

Gamon, M., Aue, A., CorSton-Oliver, S., & Ringger, E. (2005). Pulse: Mining customer opinions from free text. *International Symposium on Intelligent Data Analysis*, *3646*, 121–132.

Gonzalez-Polledo, E., & Tarr, J. (2016). The thing about pain: The remaking of illness narratives in chronic pain expressions on social media. *New Media & Society*, *18*(8), 1455–1472.

Gordon, S. L. (1981). The sociology of sentiments and emotions. In M. Rosenberg & R. H. Turner (Eds.), *Social psychology: Sociological perspectives* (pp. 562–592). New York: Basic Books.

Grandey, A. A. (2000). Emotional regulation in the workplace: A new way to conceptualize emotional labor. *Journal of Occupational Health Psychology*, *5*(1), 95–110.

Jerolmack, C., & Khan, S. (2014). Talk is cheap: Ethnography and the attitudinal fallacy. *Sociological Methods and Research*, *43*(2), 178–209.

Jobst, N. (2021). *Number of social network users in South Korea from 2017 to 2026 (in millions)*. Hamburg: Statista. Retrieved from www.statista.com/statistics/247943/number-of-social-network-users-in-south-korea/

Lacetera, N., Macis, M., & Mele, A. (2016). Viral altruism? Charitable giving and social contagion in online networks. *Sociological Science*, Article 3.

Lai, T. (2021). *Number of social network users in China from 2017 to 2020 with a forecast until 2026*. Hamburg: Statista. Retrieved from www.statista.com/statistics/277586/number-of-social-network-users-in-china/

Landy, R., Cameron, C., Au, A., Cameron, D., O'Brien, K., Robrigado, K., Baxter, L., Cockburn, L., O'Hearn, S., Oliver, B., & Nixon, S. (2016). Educational strategies to enhance reflexivity among clinicians and health professional students: A scoping study. *Forum Qualitative Sozialforschung/Forum: Qualitative Social Research*, *17*(3), Article 14.

Lieberman, M. A., & Goldstein, B. A. (2006). Not all negative emotions are equal: The role of emotional expression in online support groups for women with breast cancer. *Psycho-Oncology*, *15*(2), 160–168.

Litt, E. (2012). *Knock, Knock*. Who's there? The imagined audience. *Journal of Broadcasting & Electronic Media*, *56*(3), 330–345.

Marwick, A. E., & boyd, d. (2010). I tweet honestly, I tweet passionately: Twitter users, context collapse, and the imagined audience. *New Media Society*, *13*(1), 1–20.

Onnela, J. P., & Reed-Tsochas, F. (2010). Spontaneous emergence of social influence in online systems. *Proceedings of the National Academy of Sciences of USA*, *107*, 18375–18380.

Ritzer, G., & Jurgenson, N. (2010). Production, consumption, prosumption: The nature of capitalism in the age of the digital 'prosumer'. *Journal of Consumer Culture*, *10*(1), 13–36.

Robinson, L. (2007). The cyberself: The self-ing project goes online, symbolic interaction in the digital age. *New Media & Society*, *9*(1), 93–110.

Simmel, G. (1976). The metropolis and mental life. In K. Wolff (Ed.), *The sociology of Georg Simmel*. New York: Free Press. (Original work published 1903)

Statista Research Department. (2021). *Number of social media users in Japan from 2017 to 2020 with a forecast until 2026 (in millions)*. Hamburg: Statista. Retrieved from www.statista.com/statistics/278994/number-of-social-network-users-in-japan/

Szell, M., Lambiotte, R., & Turner, S. (2010) Multirelational organization of large-scale social networks in an online world. *Proceedings of the National Academy of Sciences of USA*, *107*, 13636–13641.

Thoits, P. (1989). The sociology of emotions. *Annual Review of Sociology*, *15*, 317–342.

Tian, X. (2017). Embodied versus disembodied information: How online artifacts influence offline interpersonal interactions. *Symbolic Interaction*, *40*(2), 190–211.

Tian, X., & Menchik, D. A. (2016). On violating one's own privacy: N-adic utterances and inadvertent disclosures in online venues. *Communication and Information Technologies Annual Studies in Communication*, *11*, 3–30.

Vaccaro, C. A., Schrock, D. P., & McCabe, J. M. (2011). Managing emotional manhood: Fighting and fostering fear in mixed martial arts. *Social Psychology Quarterly*, *74*(4), 414–437.

Conclusion

Mental Health in a New Modernity of Disenfranchisement and Risk

Toward a New Modernity: Regional Pressures on Mental Health

As Chapter 1 discussed, individual experiences of mental health are patterned by social structures, of which culture is one of the most prominent yet neglected. These cultural influences are compounded by the existence of new political and economic transformations. China, Japan, and South Korea have all evinced a rush to development culminating in unprecedented economic turmoil. These tectonic shifts in East Asia have heralded the advent of a new modernity: a second modernity arising out of a crumbling first modernity that have made ubiquitous a sense of risk.

Risk originates in a general sense of insecurity about one's ability to survive. Zygmunt Bauman called this liquid fear (Bauman, 2006, 2007) – not knowing where danger would strike next, yet keenly aware of the omnipresent potential for danger, inspiring a permanent state of fear. Risk has shifted its form over the years. In the premodern world, risk had to do with religion, weather, and violence. The greatest sources of risk to survival then were whether one would be swept away by a landslide or flood. With the rapid development of East Asia, the ontological profile of risk changed to focus more on deteriorating political and economic conditions (Beck, 1992a, 1992b; Giddens, 1990).

Scholars have generated interesting discussions linking risk society and reflexive modernization to the very real, pressing issues of inequality (Giddens, 2009; Stern, 2007). This theoretical focus allows us to consider how different, especially non-Western, regions develop and the challenges that have arisen as a result (Beck, 2009; Beck & Grande, 2007; Beck & Grande, 2010, p. 412). Although nuclear disaster, climate change, and terrorism are recognized as threatening in East Asia, they are also associated with little probability of occurrence (Han & Shim, 2010). In East Asia, there exist social risks that concern the preservation of one's existence in terms of their social well-being.

Dynamics of social interactions in East Asia are governed by a set of normative forces uncommon to Western civilization: forces rooted

DOI:10.4324/9781003308720-7

in collectivization, or a focus on preserving the interests of the collective and shaping oneself to fit into it. This dynamic goes beyond mere conformity, as efforts to preserve the interests of one's social group are undertaken for expressive, more than instrumental, reasons concerning preservation of the family's interests above individual ones within a collectivistic culture.

As Chapters 2, 3, and 4 described, these normative dynamics are captured in the norms of social exchange inherent in the purpose network behavior (Chang, 2011) or instrumental-level ties, ways of networking and ways of thinking about networking decisions unique to East Asians. The normative component enters into even dyadic contexts by invoking reputational qualities, such as tie-strength, trust, and esteem (Barbalet, 2017), but also normative qualities, such as face. How face is created and destroyed, however, depends on collectively decided values, beliefs, and expectations.

These demands to serve the larger social unit are what lead to pressures for achievement and, by extension, new risks for economic well-being as well as existential and mental health risks. Cultural beliefs that push individuals toward maintaining the status quo, familial honor, and status all depend a great deal on individual status and achievement, as previous chapters show. Indeed, traditions can both be barriers to development and enrich and inform one's identity (Giddens, 1995, p. 83; Han & Shim, 2010). We observed in previous chapters, for instance, how cultural traditions matter tremendously for individual decision-making when it comes to their mental health and interactions across the physician-patient divide, primarily because of their identity.

East Asian cultures are uniquely collectivistic. The metrics for individual worth become based on the success of the family rather than one's own achievements, as these cultures emphasize the prominence of the family's needs over those of its individual members. Consequently, their autonomy erodes, giving rise to behaviors that further compromise this autonomy, committing acts for the family rather than for the self per obligations to maintain a sense of filial piety. It renders the individual more susceptible to indoctrination by family traditions, such as satisfying their desires for improved social standing. This opens up pathways to a variety of social risks in different types of traditional pressures.

The kinds of achievement that count toward the imaginary rubric of success that East Asian cultures espouse are various. For one, there is marital achievement. People within East Asian cultures are beholden to traditional expectations about marrying someone of the opposite gender, having children, and starting a nuclear family of their own as their ancestors did in the past (Yeung et al., 2018). In East Asia, people and especially women are pressured to be married or be branded "old maids" who jeopardize the family's face and risk losing their esteem among members of kinship and social networks. Customs in East Asia also mandate parents not only take care of their children but supervise their sexuality, such that unmarried women who "live alone without parental protection and supervision risk the derogatory reputation of having loose sexual morals" (Song, 2010, p. 132).

Young, single women report being harassed by neighbors and coworkers for their single lifestyle, being persuaded to abandon their single lifestyle, patronized for their solitude, and recommended potential partners. Deviance from traditionalized conceptions of normality earns stigmatized brands of immaturity or curses. Like those at risk of mental health disorders, which are seen as curses, people who do not conform to expectations of a heterosexual, married, nuclear family are conceived as defective.

Second, there is occupational achievement. This most clearly maps onto the imperative for attaining status in East Asian cultures, where income and occupational prestige unsurprisingly constitute pathways to upward mobility, better evaluation by peers, and greater life chances altogether (Tsai et al., 2016).

Yet, these two forms of achievement – and survival itself – are under threat in contemporary East Asia under patterns of inequality and socioeconomic disenfranchisement gaining force in the region.

Real wages have been stagnating relative to inflation over the past 20 years (Figure 7.1). We see some heterogeneity here. China demonstrates exceptional average real wage growth, even after accounting for inflation, coming out to about 39% annualized growth during this period. Japan and South Korea noticeably lag far behind. Japan's average real wages stagnated for the entire period, and those of South Korea notched mild growth at about 2% annually.

For all three countries, however, costs of living are rising. In addition to inflation, real estate prices have been skyrocketing in the housing sector, which is privatized in East Asia. Let us consider a ratio that compares the average house price to average household disposable income and apply it to major metropolises in the three nations. Ideally, the standard should be 2.6, meaning it should take a household 2.6 years of their income to pay off a mortgage. Using data from Oxford Economics, a report by the private Canadian investment management firm Colliers found that the ratio is 24.6 in Beijing, 20.3 in Shanghai, 11 in Tokyo, and 17.9 in Seoul, as of 2021 (Lau, 2021). These ratios place them far ahead of every other city in the world, eclipsing even New York and Toronto. For these major cities that are often taken to represent their respective nations, the growth in wages is commensurate with, if not eclipsed by, the growth in property prices.

That costs of living are rising is felt on an everyday level. Let us consider the relative poverty rate, or the proportion of people who earn less

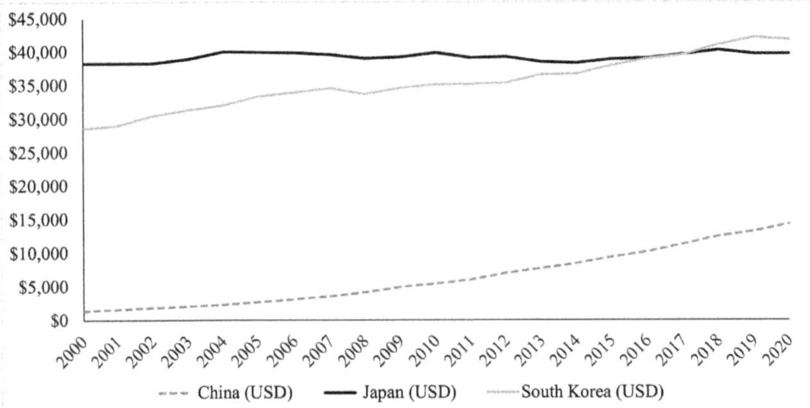

Figure 7.1 Average annual real wages (inflation-adjusted) in China, Japan, and South Korea.

Sources: Author's calculations using data from Organisation for Economic Co-operation and Development (2022)

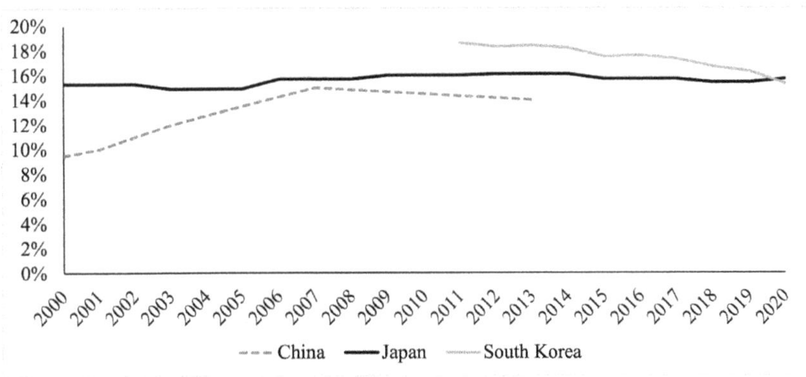

Figure 7.2 Relative poverty rates in China, Japan, and South Korea.

Sources: Author's calculations using Statista data (Huang, 2020; Statista Research Department, 2022; Yoon, 2022) and Gustafsson and Sai (2020)

than a certain (usually 50%) percentage of the median income in a general population based on available data (Figure 7.2).

Japan hovered around 16% for the past 20 years as of 2020, and South Korea mildly declined from 19% to 16% during the same period. This places them a head and shoulders above the 11.7% average for other developed nations in the Organisation for Economic Co-operation and Development (OECD). China exhibited the lowest, but which was still around 14% as of 2013, the last available data point.

These economic pressures are being felt on a household level, with family sizes shrinking drastically over time. Individuals earning less and less in wages relative to rising costs are naturally feeling less prepared and inclined to start families or have children. The age of marriage is rising in East Asia, and nearly a third of adults are still single at age 40 (Yeung et al., 2018). Additionally, we see declining birth rates in China, Japan, and South Korea (Figure 7.3).

Figure 7.4 zooms out to show the extent of this demographic trend in society at large. What is most striking is how the birth rate per 1,000 people in China, Japan, and South Korea are not only shrinking but are being eclipsed by the death rate per 1,000 people. Though Japan crossed that point as early as in 2005, South Korea just passed this pivotal moment in 2020 and China looks poised to do the same. Put differently, people in these societies do not have sufficient incentive to have (multiple) children, a large part owing to the costs of childrearing and rising costs of living in general. Compared to the death rate in these societies, we see that more members of society are dying than are being created (by birth or by immigration).

These trajectories of inequality and socioeconomic disenfranchisement compound cultural pressures on mental health. Mental health closely tails these trends, evinced by the growing incidence and prevalence of mental health illnesses over the past 20 years discussed in Chapters 1 and 2.

East Asian governments must act preemptively to revitalize their ailing mental health and social resources that are woefully unprepared for the coming crisis after COVID-19. In the short-term, this means providing more funding to hire more social workers and replenish their diminishing ranks and setting up a permanent unit to oversee

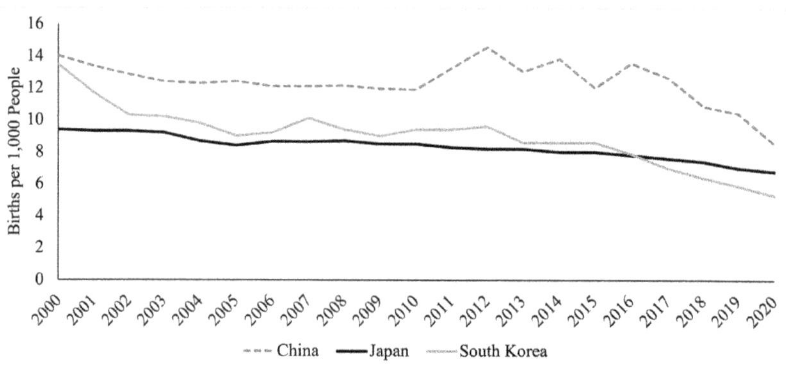

Figure 7.3 Birth rates (number of births per 1,000 people) in China, Japan, and South Korea.

Source: The World Bank (2022a)

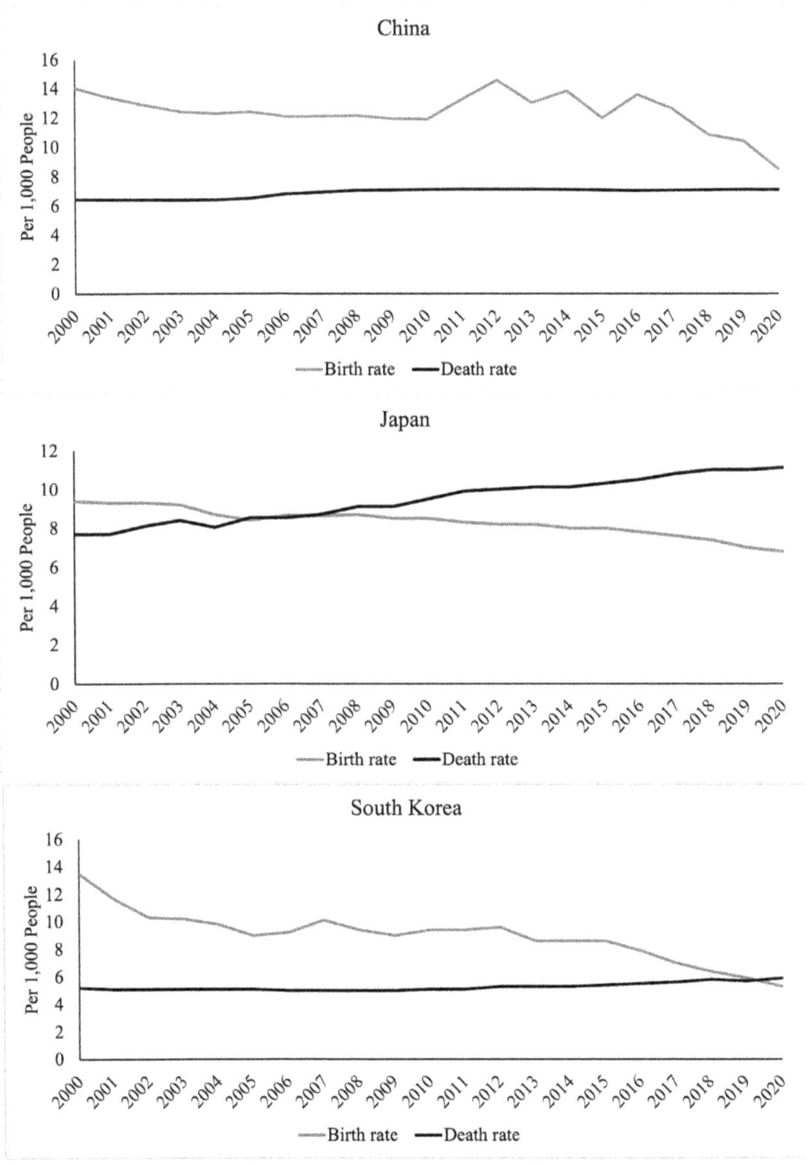

Figure 7.4 Birth and death rates compared in China, Japan, and South Korea.
Source: Author's calculations using data from the World Bank (2022a, 2022b)

population mental health within their health departments. In the long term, this means developing more sustainable workplace policies and equitable wage laws to lower inequality – and enforcing these new regulations.

Imagining a Better Future

Cultural Change

Analyzing mental health through a cultural lens reveals the need for more accommodating culture-specific services that assuage stress and its sources among East Asian immigrants and which bolster their personal coping resources. If the pandemic has taught us anything, it is that it pays to be prepared. The pandemic has exacerbated many of the mental health issues faced by residents of the region.

Cultural beliefs can be a boon for mental health coping, such as when embeddedness turbocharges one's ability to obtain social support, but those that stigmatize mental health present roadblocks for individuals experiencing mental illnesses. How do these cultural beliefs change?

Sociologically, the answer lies in facilitating generational change. Stephen Vaisey and Omar Lizardo (2016) examine the durability of cultural objects over a 30-year period in a panel study over time. They find that core attitudes to do with values and morality tend to shift by being socialized into these new attitudes early in life. Such attitudes are like those toward mental health, including attitudes toward

> civil liberties and tolerance (Bryson, 1996), various opinions regarding sexuality and gender roles (Baker, 2010), attitudes toward racial minorities and interracial marriage (Firebaugh & Davis, 1988), ideas as to whether the bible is the word of God, along with membership in traditional organizations such as veteran associations and fraternal groups (Putnam, 2001), and gun ownership (Cohen & Nisbett, 1994).
>
> (Vaisey & Lizardo, 2016, p. 7)

Thus, we might reasonably expect that cultural beliefs toward mental health will change most powerfully and visibly across generations. We might also expedite this process by increasing the opportunities for children to be socialized into friendly attitudes toward mental health. This includes incorporating new educational material in schools about the subject of mental health. Given the uptake of mental health as a subject in North American cultures, doing so might serve as an exercise of cross-cultural and current affairs education.

There is appetite for educational reform in this respect, lurking thinly beneath the surface. I wrote an opinion about mental health in Hong Kong in the *South China Morning Post* in 2017. Within a year and without any advertisement, it was incorporated into reading comprehension pamphlets across secondary schools in Hong Kong. As an extension of that, I propose several truths about mental health be built into educational material in East Asian cultures.

Mental Health Problems Are the Product of Our Circumstances; and Circumstances Are Part of Being Human

Even among doctors, healthcare professionals, and scholars, mental health problems are costumed in the language of jagged teeth and bloodshot eyes, marks of a proud beast to be conquered. "Our demons." "Things we must 'fight' together."

This is wrong. We must not let ourselves drown in the fog of a war that will only bloody us in a fight against ourselves. Mental health can be elusive and its problems can be frightening. But they are not so alien, so unsolvable, and so evil as demons. Thinking that they are pushes their victims further away from us, and into the shoes of crazies, druggies, and bad examples of how to end up – unwanted labels they are forced to live with.

More than "fighting" them, we have to lay them to rest. They are things to be untangled and understood from within the unique, winding, and sometimes crooked parts of life that some of us are not able to leave, but which all of us have gone through. A person who makes an island out of his room because of depression, severed from a continent of others, is an individual's story – often dismissed as a social hermit with poor communication skills. But encountering challenges specific to our values, our histories, our experiences is a fundamentally human story, one whose pages in which we are all written. Who can say they never faced such a problem or even several at the same time?

When we demonize mental health problems, we make their victims into aliens we should lock up out of sight. The surge of institutionalization in asylums during periods when mental health problems were most stigmatized offers a harrowing reminder of this reality. But likewise, when we humanize mental health problems, we humanize their victims into fellow people coming from real places who just need some help. And only by doing so can we salvage the person from the stigma of their circumstances and reignite the right to well-being in our march toward a better society.

Mental Health Is a Social Mirror

Mental health consequences are almost exclusively discussed in terms of often-cited, but largely unpacked statistics on depression, anxiety, and other problems. Yet, the scope of mental health reaches far beyond the individualistic picture these statistics paint, reflecting processes taken root in larger communities.

Mental health problems happen to a single person. But its causes are manifold and connected across the social, cultural, political, economic layers of social reality that enshroud us. High rates of drug abuse and delinquent behavior within a neighborhood actually tell captivating stories of family norms in street culture, of inadequate services for lower socioeconomic classes, of lack of resources being invested in schools and educational role models, of people clawing at a wall only because they have been pushed against it for too long.

Mental health statistics do not just tell us where the trees are planted, but the taste of their soil; not just where the problems are, but why. And the problems themselves reveal poignant narratives about broader changes in our communities.

Preserving Mental Health Is a Human Value, Inseparable From the Right to Well-being

Mental health is not the violence of a mad person, neither is it born of a will to bring about chaos and evil. It is someone flailing their arms because water rises above them in a closed room. Only this time, we can see their arms, but not the water. We must stop ourselves from judging symptoms without understanding causes.

Make no mistake. Mental health problems are not idle symptoms of self-pity and victimhood; they are products of things that are inevitable as humans in society. They unravel to voice details about the circumstances common to our own lives, to our communities, and to humanity itself. And as members of a family, a community, and shared humanity, we must work from this ethical base to see mental health with the same empathy and legitimacy as physical health problems. Only by doing so can we improve life for all in our own society and beyond.

Policy Change

Workplace Policies

The three truths described prior can be incorporated into the substance of workplace policy discussions as well. We see some initiative on this front in China, with the government cracking down on the infamous nine-nine-six culture in its information technology sector. As discussed in Chapter 1, high rates of burnout were commonplace in the sector and in workplaces more broadly in East Asia. Work is valorized as a form of achievement, striving, and maturity the same way that mental health does not. People are also pressed to work overtime and take on multiple jobs as real wages continue to stagnate with respect to inflation (Figure 7.1) and costs of living, most notably real estate prices, continue to surge.

Introducing new policies to restrict the number of hours that people work is a start, but even more pressing is a set of policies to ameliorate the economic pressures building up in the general population. If people cannot afford to purchase a home, people will naturally seek a second job even if their hours for their first jobs are restricted.

Workplace policy reform might also include expanding existing health benefits. Today, employment policies in East Asia do not adequately cover mental health needs. They mostly focus on physical health needs, leaving out provision for services such as counseling. Doing so would give people the space to be weak: to let them feel and talk and trust in the potential for help. Demons, enemies, and curses are not killing people. We are. When we see someone struggle, whether it is just taking a single gasp for air or thrashing their arms like a marionette in wild dance, we ought to think of the ocean that we cannot see crashing against their skin – and reach out.

Real Estate Market Policies

Governments ought to consider reining in their domestic real estate markets. Affordable housing is becoming an Achilles' heel in global cities worldwide, but nowhere more so than East Asia. Housing prices and living costs that continue to rise in the region are juxtaposed with stagnating wages and stark socioeconomic inequality. Now more than ever, resolving the housing crisis is a matter of national security (Ng et al., 2019).

We are running out of time. The housing situation in East Asian cities is rapidly approaching a flashpoint. According to the 2020 Global Real Estate Bubble Index report released last week by the Union Bank of Switzerland (2020), the risk level of a real estate bubble is highest in world-class cities in East Asia, topped by Hong Kong, Tokyo, Shanghai, and Seoul.

To understand how to solve the housing crisis, we must first understand its origins. The regional housing crisis is not actually rooted in the issue of land supply but was created by and continues to thrive because of privatization. Let us consider the case of Hong Kong.

First, housing supply is not actually *directly* linked to land supply. How the present system works is the Hong Kong government regularly disposes an amount of land for residential purposes through public auction, tender, and private treaty grants. This is called land supply. But before this land is converted into fully constructed residential homes or housing supply, it first enters the *land bank* of private developers. A land bank is the total amount of land held and sites under construction by a developer at any given time.

The land bank step between land supply and housing supply is key. Contrary to popular depiction, land supply is not the bottleneck for new housing supply, because Hong Kong developers do not often increase their land bank to restock the land they use to build residential homes.

Rather, Hong Kong developers' construction decisions are not so much motivated by need but by profit. Research on the Hong Kong housing market shows a historical tendency for developers to artificially restrict the number of houses they construct and to time their construction based on peak buying seasons and when the economy is more bullish (Lai & Wang, 1999; Leung et al., 2020).

Furthermore, because Hong Kong residential housing policies measure residential density by strict plot ratios that restrict the gross floor area for construction, developers actually have less incentive to redevelop areas – further limiting the housing supply they produce. Simultaneously, they can easily adjust their land banks to absorb any increase in land supply from the government.

Second, the housing market in Hong Kong has essentially become an oligopoly run by for-profit firms. According to a 2020 research article on the Hong Kong housing market in *Economic and Political Studies* (Leung et al., 2020), the share of the residential housing market in Hong Kong owned by for-profit developers has grown from 70% to a whopping 90% from 1995 to 2017. The growing disconnection between a laissez-faire government and public affairs has been exacerbated by Carrie Lam's long-standing commitment to non-intervention in the private sector.

For instance, after the 2010 collapse of a dilapidated building caused deaths during her tenure as Secretary of Development, Lam infamously washed her hands off the issue and declared that "at the end of the day, the responsibility to maintain buildings rests with the owners" (Lam, 2010). Thus, deference to the private sector is also why Hong Kong's "land sharing" scheme proposing to tap into private developers' reserves has been met with little demand and weak reception (Cheng, 2020).

Third, although the Hong Kong government derives over a fifth of its yearly revenue from land premiums and real estate taxes according to the 2020–2021 budget (Chan, 2020), its public expenditure on housing has fallen far behind over time. An August 2020 report by the Transport and Housing Bureau (2020) shows that the trajectory of housing expenditure has edged downward from around 5.2% of the government's total public expenditure in 2009 to a meager 5% by 2020.

Counterpart in Japan and South Korea face a similar problem. Housing developers find loopholes to advance their development of urban sprawl with less regulatory oversight. Developers lobby, often successfully, for deregulation in real estate development, gaining the ability to develop with less regard for zoning, with fewer space constraints such as a minimum size of a unit, and with fewer height constraints such as how high an apartment can be (Sorensen, 2011). In Japan, such deregulation eventually culminated in the abdication of legal authority to regulate land use from the central government to local governments.

Thus, the privatization of the housing sector has shifted too much leverage to for-profit developers. More than a chisel to carve out piecemeal efforts like rent caps or providing more land to developers, the government needs a battering ram to tackle the privatization at the heart of the housing crisis and seize greater direct control of the housing market.

Regional governments have an arsenal of legal powers at its disposal to remove the froth and excess from its housing market bubble. In Hong Kong, this takes the form of the Lands Resumption Ordinance, specifically Section 3, which reserves the Chief Executive's power to order the resumption of any land for a public purpose. While critics may damn this move as detrimental to the local business environment, a closer look at the West shows this is not the case. Resumption, called expropriation in the West, is essentially when the government mandates the sale of private property for use toward public good. In many G7 countries, such as Canada and the United States, it is a governmental right that is already regularly invoked to support infrastructure projects requiring land.

China is perhaps the nation with the most amount of coverage about its liberal use of land expropriation. Through a spatial analysis of land conflicts in China, Qiaowei Lin and colleagues (2018) find that though land conflicts may arise when the government attempts to expropriate land, conflicts eventually decrease in the population with sufficient compensation.

Another option for governments is consolidating a sovereign wealth fund like Singapore's Temasek Holdings. A state-owned holding company for investment into key sectors like housing, communications, and social amenities could be a powerful way to wrestle back critical leverage without disrupting the overall business environment. Just as important, a sovereign wealth fund could provide new jobs, invest in local firms to assist their internationalization, as well as secure the long-term financial stability of the domestic economy and insure it from financial crises (Huat, 2016).

As Machiavelli once wrote, good governance and order rely not only on strong laws to protect the people's well-being but on strong arms to guard them, even when the threat comes from within. Given how multifaceted the roots of regional socioeconomic pressures truly are, governments need a swift, decisive, and forceful approach to reverse the privatization that has overstepped its boundaries in their territory – or be overwhelmed once more by the human, social, and political costs of prolonged inequality and public unrest. Furthermore, governments have ample room to consider employment and educational policy reforms to broaden exposure to the subject of mental health and reduce misinformation surrounding mental illnesses.

These sets of reforms will likely reverse some of the stigmatization and, even if not within a single generation, will sow the seeds for cultural and socioeconomic change to improve mental health and quality of life in future generations. At that time, we may well learn to care for someone before they become a headline, to have sympathy for the living before they become the dead.

References

Baker, W. (2010). The duality of american moral culture. In S. Hitlin & S. Vaisey (Eds.), *Handbook of the sociology of morality* (pp. 255–274). New York: Springer.
Barbalet, J. (2017). Dyadic characteristics of Guanxi and their consequences. *Journal for the Theory of Social Behaviour*, *47*(3), 332–347.
Bauman, Z. (2006). *Liquid fear*. Cambridge: Polity Press.
Bauman, Z. (2007). *Liquid times: Living in an age of uncertainty*. Cambridge: Polity Press.
Beck, U. (1992a). Risk society: Towards a new modernity. London: SAGE.
Beck, U. (1992b). From industrial society to the risk society: Questions of survival, social structure and ecological enlightenment. *Theory, Culture & Society*, *9*, 97–123.
Beck, U. (2009). *World at risk*. Cambridge: Polity Press.
Beck, U., & Grande, E. (2007). *Cosmopolitan Europe*. Cambridge: Polity Press.
Beck, U., & Grande, E. (2010). Varieties of second modernity: The cosmopolitan turn in social and political theory and research. *British Journal of Sociology*, *61*(3), 409–443.
Bryson, B. (1996). "Anything but heavy metal": Symbolic exclusion and musical dislikes. *American Sociological Review*, *61*(5), 884–899.
Chan, P. (2020). *The 2020–2021 budget*. HKSAR: Government of the Hong Kong Special Administrative Region. Retrieved from www.budget.gov.hk/2020/eng/pdf/e_budget_speech_2020-21.pdf
Chang, K. (2011). A path to understanding *Guanxi* in China's transitional economy: Variations on network behavior. *Sociological Theory*, *29*(4), 315–339.
Cheng, L. (2020). Hong Kong developers ignore scheme to boost land supply for housing by converting private reserves in New Territories. *South China Morning Post*. Retrieved from www.scmp.com/news/hong-kong/society/article/3102257/hong-kong-developers-ignore-scheme-boost-land-supply-housing
Cohen, D., & Nisbett, R. E. (1994). Self-protection and the culture of honor: Explaining southern violence. *Personality & Social Psychology Bulletin*, *20*(5), 551–567.
Firebaugh, G., & Davis, K. E. (1988). Trends in antiblack prejudice, 1972–1984: Region and cohort effects. *American Journal of Sociology*, *94*(2), 251–272.
Giddens, A. (1990). *Consequences of modernity*. Redwood City, CA: Stanford University Press.
Giddens, A. (1995). Living in a post-traditional society. In U. Beck, A. Giddens, & S. Lash (Eds.), *Reflexive modernization* (pp. 56–109). Stanford, CA: Stanford University Press.
Giddens, A. (2009). *The politics of climate change*. Cambridge: Polity Press.

Gustafsson, B., & Sai, D. (2020). Growing into relative income poverty: Urban China, 1988–2013. *Social Indicators Research*, *147*(1), 73–94.
Han, S. J., & Shim, Y. H. (2010). Redefining second modernity for east-Asia: A critical assessment. *British Journal of Sociology*, *61*(3), 465–489.
Huang, E. (2020, July 2). Japan's middle class is 'disappearing' as poverty rises, warns economist. *CNBC News*. Retrieved from www.cnbc.com/2020/07/03/japans-middle-class-is-disappearing-as-poverty-rises-warns-economist.html
Huat, C. B. (2016). State-owned enterprises, state capitalism and social distribution in Singapore. *The Pacific Review*, *29*(4), 499–521.
Lai, N., & Wang, K. (1999). Land-supply restrictions, developer strategies and housing policies: The case in Hong Kong. *International Real Estate Review*, *2*(1), 143–159.
Lam, C. (2010, January 30). *Secretary for development speaks about building collapse*. HKSAR: Development Bureau, Government of the Hong Kong Special Administrative Region.
Lau, C. K. (2021). *Do high residential prices and the Evergrande episode signal falling China property values?* Toronto: Colliers. Retrieved from www.colliers.com/en-xa/news/blog-cvas-do-high-residential-prices-and-evergrande-episode-signal-falling-china-property-values
Leung, C. K. Y., Ng, J. C. Y., & Tang, E. C. H. (2020). What do we know about housing supply? The case of Hong Kong SAR. *Economic and Political Studies*, *8*(1), 6–20.
Lin, Q., Tan, S., Zhang, L., Wang, S., Wei, C., & Li, Y. (2018). Conflicts of land expropriation in China during 2006–2016: An overview and its spatio-temporal characteristics. *Land Use Policy*, *76*, 246–251.
Ng, J., Cheung, G., & Tsang, D. (2019). Hong Kong policy address key takeaways: Leader Carrie Lam homes in on housing 'grievances' and unveils cash sweeteners in bid to rescue city from brink. *South China Morning Post*. Retrieved from www.scmp.com/news/hong-kong/politics/article/3033174/policy-address-key-takeaways-carrie-lam-homes-housing
Organisation for Economic Co-operation and Development. (2022). *Average annual wages*. Paris: Organisation for Economic Co-operation and Development. https://stats.oecd.org/index.aspx?DataSetCode=AV_AN_WAGE
Putnam, R. D. (2001). *Bowling alone: The collapse and revival of American community*. New York: Simon & Schuster.
Song, J. (2010). 'A room of one's own': The meaning of spatial autonomy for unmarried women in neoliberal South Korea. *Gender, Place & Culture*, *17*(2), 131–149.
Sorensen, A. (2011). Evolving property rights in Japan: Patterns and logics of change. *Urban Studies*, *48*(3), 471–491.
Statista Research Department. (2022). *Poverty rate Japan 1991–2018*. Hamburg: Statista. Retrieved from www.statista.com/statistics/1172622/japan-poverty-rate/
Stern, N. (2007). *The economics of climate change: The stern report*. Cambridge: Cambridge University Press.
The World Bank. (2022a). *Birth rate, crude (per 1,000 people)*. Washington, DC: Author. Retrieved from https://data.worldbank.org/indicator/SP.DYN.CBRT.IN

The World Bank. (2022b). *Death rate, crude (per 1,000 people)*. Washington, DC: Author. Retrieved from https://data.worldbank.org/indicator/SP.DYN.CDRT.IN

Transport and Housing Bureau. (2020). *Housing in figures 2020*. HKSAR: Transport and Housing Bureau, Government of the Hong Kong Special Administrative Region. Retrieved from www.thb.gov.hk/eng/psp/publications/housing/HIF2020.pdf

Tsai, M. C., Nitta, M., Kim, S. W., & Wang, W. (2016). Working overtime in East Asia: Convergence or divergence? *Journal of Contemporary Asia*, *46*(4), 700–722.

Union Bank of Switzerland. (2020). *UBS global real estate bubble index 2020*. Zurich: Union Bank of Switzerland, Chief Investment Office.

Vaisey, S., & Lizardo, O. (2016). Cultural fragmentation or acquired dispositions? A new approach to accounting for patterns of cultural change. *Socius*, 2, 1–15.

Yeung, W. J. J., Desai, S., & Jones, G. W. (2018). Families in southeast and South Asia. *Annual Review of Sociology*, *44*, 469–495.

Yoon, L. (2022). *Relative poverty rate South Korea 2011–2020*. Hamburg: Statista. Retrieved from www.statista.com/statistics/1225832/south-korea-realative-poverty-rate/#:~:text=In%202020%2C%20the%20relative%20poverty,fallen%20steadily%20in%20recent%20years

Appendix
Data and Methods

This monograph draws on a variety of primary and secondary data sources.

Statistical Data

All datasets that this monograph draws from were publicly available and open access. I draw in particular on the World Health Organization's 2019 Global Burden of Disease Study (GBDS) with a focus on mental health, jointly produced by the Institute of Health Metrics and Evaluation. GBDS data is released regularly, is statistically representative of the general population, and covers populations in virtually every nation. For the purposes of this book, I focus on China, Japan, and South Korea.

The epidemiological measures captured in the dataset include the number of deaths in the population, number of disability-adjusted years of life (DALYs) in the population, number of years of life lost (YLLs) in the population, number of years lived with disability (YLDs) in the population, total number of cases in the population, number new of cases in the population, prevalence rate, and incidence rate. The mental health spectrum covered in the dataset was broad, but I focus on the most prevalent, namely those in Figure 1. For illustrative purposes, I also collated these measures wherever appropriate and indicated as such, such as the prevalence of drug use and of alcohol use into a single measure of substance abuse more broadly.

I draw also on Statista data on social media use in the general population in China, Japan, and South Korea, which is built by triangulating various sources that include government data and Statista market researchers. Statista is a world-renowned database company that focuses on generating market and consumer data worldwide in similar fashion to Bloomberg.

I further draw on wage data and demographic trend data from the Organisation for Economic Co-operation and Development and the World Bank, as well as from the 2012 Japanese General Social Survey (JGSS) (JGSS Research Center, Osaka University of Commerce, 2016) and 2017 Chinese General Social Survey (CGSS) (National Natural Science Foundation of China, 2017), both of which are statistically representative datasets on their respective nations. The JGSS is administered by the Osaka University of Commerce, and its data is archived with the Leibniz Institute for the Social Sciences. Using a probability-based multistage sampling approach, it is consisted of 4,667 respondents. The CGSS is administered by the National Natural Science Foundation of China using a regionally stratified sampling approach and consisted of 12,582 respondents in the 2017 version. Any missing data for a given measure were removed and not pictured in the final analyses presented in-text.

Case Studies

I conducted several case studies of physician-patient interactions within East Asia over the course of two years from 2017 to 2019. Robert Yin (2003) classically described the case study as a way to study a phenomenon in terms of "how" and "why" it transpires, as well as the contexts under which it does. Anthony Giddens goes on to elaborate the utility of a case study in connection to ethnography as:

> Research which is geared primarily to hermeneutic problems may be of generalized importance in so far as it serves to elucidate the nature of agents' knowledgeability, and thereby their reasons for action, across a wide range of action-contexts. Pieces of ethnographic research like . . . say, the traditional small-scale community research of fieldwork anthropology – are not in themselves generalizing studies. But they can easily become so if carried out in some numbers, so that judgements of their typicality can justifiably be made.
>
> (Giddens, 1984, p. 328)

Put differently, case studies have the analytical power to build generalizable principles to refute the status quo. We might think of this in terms of Karl Popper's falsification hypothesis (1959, pp. 1–4): to seek out observations that violate the status quo or a given hypothesis as a sort of test of its veracity. If we find the existence of just one black swan, for instance, we will no longer have grounds to say that all swans are white. This will prompt us to rethink the generalizability of a widely held idea and develop new generalizable ideas instead.

Following a similar logic of inquiry, I conducted observations of physicians interacting with their patients over two years largely through a systematic ethnography of clinics during this period. I chose seven prominent clinics or hospitals that served clients in South Korea, a highly popular destination for private medicine and medical tourism. South Korea is perhaps the largest of the three East Asian nations in attracting tourists for medical procedures on their soil, such as with over 200,000 visitors per year, the majority of which come from China (Statista Research Department, 2022).

The clinics or hospitals themselves were providers of cosmetic surgery services, but which also included reparative surgery services for health rather than aesthetic reasons, such as corrections for deviated septums or ptosis. While there, I often did not interact and mostly recorded my observations of clinician and patients as they interacted as well as within the waiting room spaces. Prior to any observation, I obtained verbal consent from all participants. In the waiting rooms, I at times engaged in field interviews or casual conversations about patients' perceptions of their private medicine services of interest.

Both forms of participant observation produce a causal way of explaining the logic behind patient and professional attitudes toward mental health, toward each other, and toward their cultural beliefs by capturing the interpretive mechanisms driving "how" and "why" these perceptions come to be (Small, 2009).

Interviews and Positionality

Twenty-four Chinese student participants were recruited from universities in Hong Kong (6 males and 18 females) using a nonrandom sampling method. The nonrandom sampling scheme was motivated by theoretical interests in obtaining the widest reach in the types of users who used social media. The data used for this chapter come from a larger project about social media use among youth in Hong Kong. Findings from the larger project show how users largely fell into two groups: frequent users who used social media apps nearly every day or detached users who used but did not interact on social media. Interestingly, findings also showed how norms of social media activity were nonetheless universally recognized, understood, and known among all users, even among detached users who rejected them.

Questions centered on their use of social media, their choices of which social networking site to use, the functions and resources they use, the ways they interact with others online, the ways they represent themselves online, comparisons between online and offline behaviors, and reflections on their and others' profiles as representations of the self. Each interview lasted around one hour, and the project ended when thematic saturation was achieved (Bowen, 2008; Jerolmack & Khan, 2014). All interviews were conducted by the author, which lasted about an hour each. Transcriptions were conducted with help from two assistants, and analyses were performed by the author.

Qualitative Analysis

I analyzed my qualitative (case study, ethnographic, and interview) data using the same analytical strategy. Adopting a theoretically flexible approach to explore themes and patterns in masses of data, I conducted thematic coding and a cross-comparative analysis of such themes (Au, 2016; Attride-Stirling, 2001; Braun & Clarke, 2006). This approach finds similarities with cross-comparative coding frameworks native to grounded theory (Charmaz, 2006). In the initial phase of open coding, I labeled and organized data into different themes. In focused coding, I found commonalities within those codes to formulate higher-level abstractions while using the most salient among them to recursively filter the data to "determine the adequacy" of such codes (ibid., p. 57). Afterward, I used axial coding to reconstruct broader theorizations about emotions, mental health, stigma, treatment, and cultural beliefs by "[linking] categories with subcategories, and [asking] how they are related" (ibid., p. 61).

In so doing, I compared cases within the same theme and across different themes to inductively and systematically push them toward higher-level theorizations that make sense of the connection between emotions and social media in the context of different social user roles, as well as cultural beliefs espoused by physicians and patients as they impinged upon their interactions and imaginations of one another and of mental health.

All names mentioned in the monograph have been changed to protect real identities.

References

Attride-Stirling, J. (2001). Thematic networks: An analytic tool for qualitative research. *Qualitative Research*, *1*(3), 385–405.

Au, A. (2016). Reconceptualizing online free spaces: A case study of the sunflower movement. *Journal of Contemporary Eastern Asia*, *15*(2), 145–161.

Bowen, G. A. (2008). Naturalistic inquiry and the saturation concept: A research note. *Qualitative Research*, *8*(1), 137–152.

Braun, V., & Clarke, V. (2006). Using thematic analysis in psychology. *Qualitative Research in Psychology*, *3*(2), 77–101.

Charmaz, K. (2006). *Constructing grounded theory: A practical guide through qualitative analysis*. Thousand Oaks, CA: SAGE.

Giddens, A. (1984). *The constitution of society: Outline of the theory of structuration*. Cambridge: Polity Press.

Jerolmack, C., & Khan, S. (2014). Talk is cheap: Ethnography and the attitudinal fallacy. *Sociological Methods and Research*, *43*(2), 178–209.

JGSS Research Center, Osaka University of Commerce. (2016). *Japanese General Social Survey 2012 (JGSS 2012)* [ZA6427 Data file Version 2.0.0]. Cologne: GESIS Data Archive. https://doi.org/10.4232/1.12604. Retrieved from https://search.gesis.org/research_data/ZA6427

National Natural Science Foundation of China. 中国综合社会调查. (2017). *Chinese general social survey 2017*. Beijing: National Natural Science Foundation of China. Retrieved from www.cnsda.org/index.php?r=projects/view&id=94525591

Popper, K. (1959). *The logic of scientific inquiry*. London: Routledge.
Small, M. L. (2009). How many cases do I need? On science and the logic of case selection in field-based research. *Ethnography*, *10*(1), 5–38.
Statista Research Department. (2022). *Medical tourism in South Korea – statistics & facts*. Hamburg: Statista. Retrieved from www.statista.com/topics/6382/medical-tourism-in-south-korea/#topicHeader__wrapper
Yin, R. K. (2003). *Case study research: Design and methods* (3rd ed.). Thousand Oaks, CA: SAGE.

Index

For Product Safety Concerns and Information please contact our EU
representative GPSR@taylorandfrancis.com
Taylor & Francis Verlag GmbH, Kaufingerstraße 24, 80331 München, Germany

www.ingramcontent.com/pod-product-compliance
Ingram Content Group UK Ltd.
Pitfield, Milton Keynes, MK11 3LW, UK
UKHW020136200926
475702UK00005B/767
* 9 7 8 1 0 3 2 3 1 0 3 7 4 *